616.9515
K832g

DETROIT PUBLIC LIBRARY

3 5674 04328187 3

DEADLY DISEASES AND EPIDEMICS

GONORRHEA

D0139823

CHANDLER PARK LIBRARY
12800 HARPER
DETROIT, MI 48213

AUG - 2006

CP

Anthrax

Campylobacteriosis

Cholera

Escherichia coli Infections

Gonorrhea

Hepatitis

Herpes

HIV/AIDS

Influenza

Lyme Disease

Mad Cow Disease (Bovine Spongiform Encephalopathy)

Malaria

Meningitis

Mononucleosis

Plague

Polio

SARS

Smallpox

Streptococcus (Group A)

Syphilis

Toxic Shock Syndrome

Tuberculosis

Typhoid Fever

West Nile Virus

DEADLY DISEASES AND EPIDEMICS

GONORRHEA

Linda Kollar
and
Brian R. Shmaefsky

CONSULTING EDITOR

The Late **I. Edward Alcamo**
Distinguished Teaching Professor of Microbiology,
SUNY Farmingdale

FOREWORD BY

David Heymann
World Health Organization

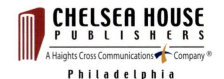

CHELSEA HOUSE
PUBLISHERS
A Haights Cross Communications ✦ Company ®

Philadelphia

COVER: *Neisseria gonorrhoeae*, the bacterium that causes gonorrhea, is shown here. This image was taken with a transmission electron microscope and is magnified 45,000 times.

Dedication
We dedicate the books in the DEADLY DISEASES AND EPIDEMICS series to Ed Alcamo, whose wit, charm, intelligence, and commitment to biology education were second to none.

CHELSEA HOUSE PUBLISHERS
VP, NEW PRODUCT DEVELOPMENT Sally Cheney
DIRECTOR OF PRODUCTION Kim Shinners
CREATIVE MANAGER Takeshi Takahashi
MANUFACTURING MANAGER Diann Grasse

Staff for Gonorrhea
EXECUTIVE EDITOR Tara Koellhoffer
ASSOCIATE EDITOR Beth Reger
EDITORIAL ASSISTANT Kuorkor Dzani
PRODUCTION EDITOR Noelle Nardone
PHOTO EDITOR Sarah Bloom
SERIES DESIGNER Terry Mallon
COVER DESIGNER Keith Trego
LAYOUT 21st Century Publishing and Communications, Inc.

©2005 by Chelsea House Publishers,
a subsidiary of Haights Cross Communications.
All rights reserved. Printed and bound in China.

A Haights Cross Communications ◥ Company ®

http://www.chelseahouse.com

First Printing

1 3 5 7 9 8 6 4 2

Library of Congress Cataloging-in-Publication Data

Kollar, Linda.
Gonorrhea / Linda Kollar and Brian Shmaefsky ; foreword by David Heymann.
  p. cm.—(Deadly diseases and epidemics)
    Includes bibliographical references and index.
  ISBN 0-7910-7593-1 (hardcover)—ISBN 0-7910-8377-2 (pbk.)
  1. Gonorrhea. I. Shmaefsky, Brian. II. Title. III. Series.
RC202.K64 2005
616.95'15—dc22

2005003284

All links and web addresses were checked and verified to be correct at the time of publication. Because of the dynamic nature of the web, some addresses and links may have changed since publication and may no longer be valid.

Table of Contents

Foreword

In the 1960s, many of the infectious diseases that had terrorized generations were tamed. After a century of advances, the leading killers of Americans both young and old were being prevented with new vaccines or cured with new medicines. The risk of death from pneumonia, tuberculosis (TB), meningitis, influenza, whooping cough, and diphtheria declined dramatically. New vaccines lifted the fear that summer would bring polio, and a global campaign was on the verge of eradicating smallpox worldwide. New pesticides like DDT cleared mosquitoes from homes and fields, thus reducing the incidence of malaria, which was present in the southern United States and which remains a leading killer of children worldwide. New technologies produced safe drinking water and removed the risk of cholera and other water-borne diseases. Science seemed unstoppable. Disease seemed destined to all but disappear.

But the euphoria of the 1960s has evaporated.

The microbes fought back. Those causing diseases like TB and malaria evolved resistance to cheap and effective drugs. The mosquito developed the ability to defuse pesticides. New diseases emerged, including AIDS, Legionnaires, and Lyme disease. And diseases which had not been seen in decades re-emerged, as the hantavirus did in the Navajo Nation in 1993. Technology itself actually created new health risks. The global transportation network, for example, meant that diseases like West Nile virus could spread beyond isolated regions and quickly become global threats. Even modern public health protections sometimes failed, as they did in 1993 in Milwaukee, Wisconsin, resulting in 400,000 cases of the digestive system illness cryptosporidiosis. And, more recently, the threat from smallpox, a disease believed to be completely eradicated, has returned along with other potential bioterrorism weapons such as anthrax.

The lesson is that the fight against infectious diseases will never end.

In our constant struggle against disease, we as individuals have a weapon that does not require vaccines or drugs, and that is the warehouse of knowledge. We learn from the history of science that "modern" beliefs can be wrong. In this series of books, for example, you will learn that diseases like syphilis were once thought to be caused by eating potatoes. The invention of the microscope set science on the right path. There are more positive lessons from history. For example, smallpox was eliminated by vaccinating everyone who had come in contact with an infected person. This "ring" approach to smallpox control is still the preferred method for confronting an outbreak, should the disease be intentionally reintroduced.

At the same time, we are constantly adding new drugs, new vaccines, and new information to the warehouse. Recently, the entire human genome was decoded. So too was the genome of the parasite that causes malaria. Perhaps by looking at the microbe and the victim through the lens of genetics we will be able to discover new ways to fight malaria, which remains the leading killer of children in many countries.

Because of advances in our understanding of such diseases as AIDS, entire new classes of anti-retroviral drugs have been developed. But resistance to all these drugs has already been detected, so we know that AIDS drug development must continue.

Education, experimentation, and the discoveries that grow out of them are the best tools to protect health. Opening this book may put you on the path of discovery. I hope so, because new vaccines, new antibiotics, new technologies, and, most importantly, new scientists are needed now more than ever if we are to remain on the winning side of this struggle against microbes.

David Heymann
Executive Director
Communicable Diseases Section
World Health Organization
Geneva, Switzerland

1

A Teen's Experience With Gonorrhea

Every year, Roger sees his family doctor for a physical exam before football season begins. This year, Roger is going to be a senior in high school, and he is looking forward to a great season as the team's starting quarterback. After enjoying himself over the summer, hanging out with friends, and dating some girls he met at the beach, he's ready to face the tough football work-outs and academic demands that await him when school starts next week.

The doctor reviews Roger's physical health and injuries since last season. Other than a sprained ankle he got playing soccer in the spring, which healed quickly, Roger has been lucky enough to remain injury-free throughout his sports career. The doctor is happy to note this. Next, the doctor asks Roger about his use of drugs and alcohol and questions whether he is sexually active. Thankful that his mother has not come with him to the appointment, Roger tells the doctor honestly that he has never used drugs, but admits that he had sex with two girls he met at the beach over the summer and used a **condom** most of the time—although there were a few instances when he forgot to use protection. This raises a red flag for the doctor. Although Roger shows no signs of any **sexually transmitted diseases** (**STDs**), the doctor recommends that he be tested for **gonorrhea** and chlamydia, two of the most common STDs in the United States. Roger is told that he can either urinate into a cup and have his urine tested or he can have the doctor take a specimen from his penis with a cotton-tipped applicator. Roger chooses the urine test and heads off to the bathroom with the specimen cup.

A few days after his visit to the doctor's office, Roger receives a phone call at home. Again grateful that his parents aren't there, he listens in disbelief as the doctor explains that his urine test has come back positive for gonorrhea. Now he realizes that he's probably going to have to tell his parents about his sexual activity—and be treated for a serious illness.

Gonorrhea is one of the oldest and best-known STDs. Caused by a **bacterium** called **Neisseria gonorrhoeae**, the disease has been described by medical experts dating as far back as 3500 B.C. The name *gonorrhea* comes from Latin, and literally means "flowing of the **gonads**," a reference to the pus that sometimes flows from the **genitourinary tract** of infected individuals (Figure 1.1). Over the past 60 years or so in the United States, gonorrhea has come to be known by a wide variety of slang names, such as "the clap," "the drips," "race-horse," and "whites." Despite its potential to cause serious problems, as recently as the 1970s, some American men actually considered getting gonorrhea a sign of manhood.

Neisseria gonorrhoeae, like other members of the Neisseriaceae family of bacteria, normally thrives in the **mucous membranes**. This particular member is limited to the genitourinary system. Because of its spherical shape, *Neisseria gonorrhoeae* is sometimes called *gonococcus*, meaning "the round bacteria of the genitals" (Figure 1.2).

Gonorrhea is almost exclusively spread through sexual contact. In men, the *Neisseria gonorrhoeae* bacteria enter the **urethra** when the penis comes in contact with infected vaginal **mucus** during sexual intercourse, or other fluids during anal intercourse. The bacteria then use special chemicals to bind to the cells of the urethra. In women, the gonorrhea-causing bacteria are generally found lining the **cervix**, urethra, and vagina. Women typically acquire gonorrhea from sexual contact with the **semen** of an infected man.

The gonorrhea bacterium can hide from the body's immune system for 7 to 14 days after a person is first infected.

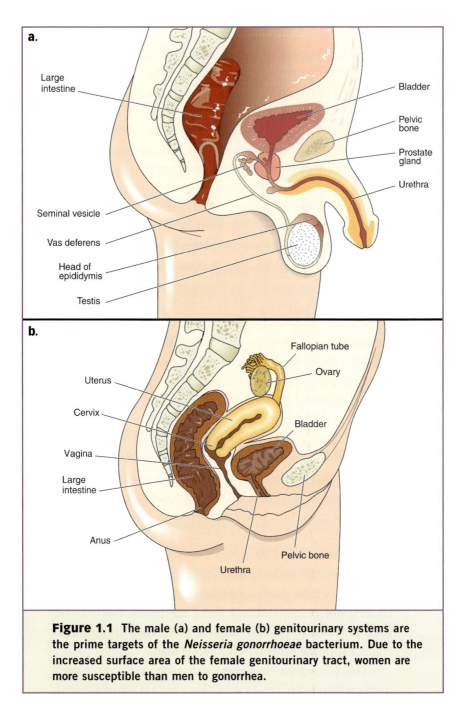

Figure 1.1 The male (a) and female (b) genitourinary systems are the prime targets of the *Neisseria gonorrhoeae* bacterium. Due to the increased surface area of the female genitourinary tract, women are more susceptible than men to gonorrhea.

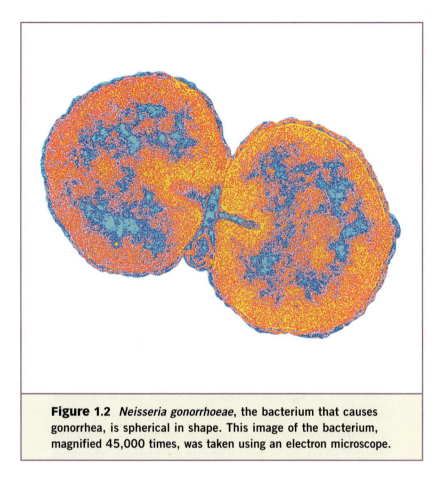

Figure 1.2 *Neisseria gonorrhoeae*, the bacterium that causes gonorrhea, is spherical in shape. This image of the bacterium, magnified 45,000 times, was taken using an electron microscope.

This is because it takes the bacteria a while to multiply to high enough concentrations to cause disease symptoms. Most often, the first sign of gonorrhea in males is slight to moderate pain during urination, although not all men (as in Roger's case) notice any symptoms. The pain that accompanies urination occurs because the urethra is being irritated by the growth and secretions of the multiplying bacteria. Females usually show no signs of disease at all in the early stages of gonorrhea infection. This is a very dangerous aspect of gonorrhea, since the infected woman who does not realize she is sick may not seek medical treatment until the disease has progressed and caused severe damage to her body, including **pelvic inflammatory disease (PID)** and possibly sterility.

Luckily for Roger, gonorrhea is one STD that can be cured. Because it is caused by a bacterium, gonorrhea can be treated with **antibiotics**, drugs that have the ability to kill different kinds of bacteria. Although both Roger and his parents were very upset about his illness, the doctor was able to give Roger an oral antibiotic prescription, and his infection was cured rapidly. Roger learned some valuable lessons from his experience—that a person may have a potentially dangerous disease and never even know it, and the importance of using condoms whenever you choose to have sex outside of a monogamous relationship with someone who is not infected with an STD.

Today, gonorrhea is very common among sexually active people between the ages of 15 and 30. The **incidence** of gonorrhea is also rapidly growing among the male homosexual and elderly populations. (*Incidence* means the number of people who contract a disease in a particular time period.) Much of this rise in the rate of gonorrhea infection is due to a disregard for **safer sex** practices. Younger people are more likely exposed to gonorrhea because of the common practice of relying on birth control (such as the pill) to reduce the "dangers" of sex. Birth control devices and methods other than condoms do *not* prevent gonorrhea.

Urban areas in almost every nation of the world are more likely than rural regions to have gonorrhea present in the population. The Centers for Disease Control and Prevention (CDC) has documented 400,000 cases of gonorrhea each year in the United States. This is significantly fewer than the number of cases there were in the 1940s before the widespread use of antibiotics and safer sex practices. However, statistics show that half of all gonorrhea cases today go undiagnosed. Based on data collected in 2002, it is believed that 650,000 people acquire the infection each year. Many people go untreated, contributing to 800,000 annual cases estimated by clinics and physicians.

The estimated numbers are gathered by interviewing people who have been diagnosed with the disease. Many of these people had sexual intercourse with a partner who was unaware that he or she had an active gonorrhea infection. Worldwide, approximately 62 million cases of gonorrhea are reported each year. Gonorrhea is unfortunately greatly underreported in many countries. That means that many more cases of the disease most likely exist, and we just do not know about them.

This book will explore the history of gonorrhea, the structure and function of the bacterium that causes it, the symptoms people usually experience and how the disease is diagnosed, and what you can do to avoid getting the disease, which, even though it is treatable, can sometimes lead to severe or even deadly complications.

2

History of Gonorrhea and Sexually Transmitted Diseases

Sexually transmitted infections such as gonorrhea are not unique to the MTV generation. Warriors in the Roman Empire, seafaring merchants of the spice routes, fur traders in the pioneer days of America, and business travelers of more modern times have all historically contracted and spread gonorrhea. The understanding and science of what are called sexually transmitted diseases (STDs), **communicable diseases** spread by sexual intercourse or genital contact, have taken many turns over the centuries. Scientific discoveries have fortunately clarified the biology and transmission of many of these diseases, including gonorrhea. In this chapter, we will look at sexually transmitted diseases, and gonorrhea in particular, examining the impact of STDs on humans over time.

COMMON SEXUALLY TRANSMITTED DISEASES

According to the Centers for Disease Control and Prevention (CDC), there are more than 15 million cases of sexually transmitted disease cases reported each year. Adolescents and young adults (ages 15 to 24) are at the greatest risk for acquiring an STD, with 3 million becoming infected each year. What are these diseases and how are they contracted?

Chlamydia

Chlamydia is caused by the bacterium *Chlamydia trachomatis* (Figure 2.1), which can severely damage a woman's reproductive organs. As with

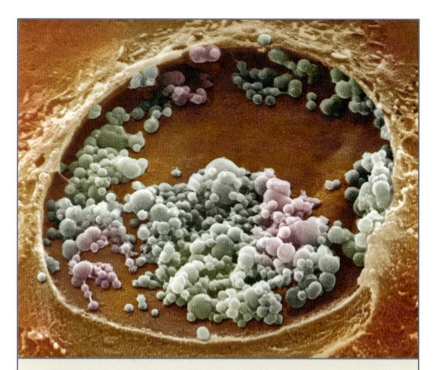

Figure 2.1 This electron micrograph shows *Chlamydia trachomatis* bacteria (green and purple spheres, colored so they can be seen more easily) in a human epithelial cell of the cervix. Chlamydia is a serious disease that often does not result in symptoms, but can cause infertility if left untreated.

gonorrhea, symptoms of chlamydia may be mild or absent in both men and women. When they do occur, symptoms include discharge from the vagina or penis and a burning sensation while urinating. Serious complications that cause irreversible damage, including infertility, can occur "silently" before the infected woman ever realizes she has a problem. Fortunately, the infection is curable with antibiotics.

Hepatitis A Virus (HAV)

Hepatitis A is a liver disease that is caused by the hepatitis A virus (HAV). It is preventable with **vaccination**. The infection is spread through oral contact with fecal matter through oral/anal sex. It is also spread through contact with infected blood, most often through sharing needles for intravenous (IV) drug use. After being infected with HAV and recovering from the illness, people develop **immunity** from reinfection but may remain contagious for the rest of their lives without ever showing symptoms of the disease. In the United States, hepatitis A can occur in many situations, ranging from isolated cases of disease to widespread **epidemics.**

Hepatitis B Virus (HBV)

Hepatitis B is also a liver disease caused by a **virus**; in this case, the hepatitis B virus (HBV). Like HAV, the infection is also preventable through vaccination. Symptoms of HBV infection include fatigue, headache, fever, hives, and swelling of the abdomen. The infection is diagnosed with a blood test. Although there is no treatment for the infection, fortunately, most people recover from the disease.

Herpes

Herpes is caused by the herpes simplex viruses type 1 (HSV-1) and type 2 (HSV-2). HSV-1 is usually associated with the cold sores and fever blisters that appear around the mouth (Figure 2.2), often when a person is under stress or hasn't been eating a healthy diet. Most people in the United States have acquired the HSV-1 virus at some point in their lives. HSV-2 is more commonly the cause of genital herpes infections. Either type of the herpes virus, however, may be sexually transmitted. If a person is infected with HSV-1 through oral sex, he or she may show symptoms of blisters in the genital region (rather than cold sores on the mouth, since the blisters appear at the site where the infection took place). Many people are infected with the virus but remain **asymptomatic**. When symptoms are present, the first outbreak of genital herpes will consist of many painful fluid-filled blisters on the vagina, cervix, penis,

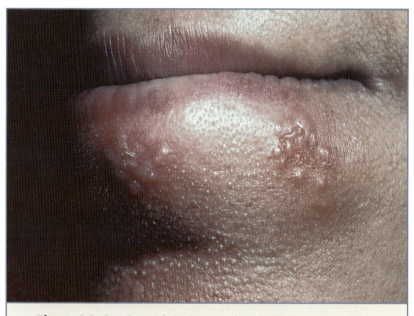

Figure 2.2 One form of the herpes virus (HSV-1) causes cold sores and fever blisters that often form around the mouth, as can be seen on the lips of the person in this photograph.

mouth, anus, or buttocks. The virus remains in the body even after the visible signs have gone away, and it can recur over and over throughout a person's life, although recurrences are generally less painful and of shorter duration. Like all viral infections, herpes has no cure. The symptoms can be relieved, however, and the number of outbreaks limited with antiviral medications.

Human Immunodeficiency Virus (HIV)

Human immunodeficiency virus (**HIV**) is the cause of acquired immunodeficiency syndrome (AIDS). After being infected, a person will usually show no symptoms for a long time—as long as 10 years or more. Once the virus has invaded the immune system, symptoms include unexplained weight loss, fatigue, fevers, night sweats, headaches, mental disorders, yeast infection in the mouth, and uncommon skin cancers. HIV attacks the cells of the immune system, and the symptoms are evidence that the person is unable to fight off **pathogens** (disease-causing organisms) that the body would normally be able to eliminate before any symptoms appear. AIDS is eventually fatal and there is no cure for the virus; however, control of the virus's progression has been achieved with antiviral medications, allowing people to live longer.

Human Papillomavirus (HPV)

Human papillomavirus (HPV) is the cause of genital warts and changes to the cells of the cervix called dysplasia. There are more than 100 strains of this virus and several types have been linked to various forms of cancer, including cervical cancer. The infection is usually asymptomatic. If genital warts develop, they are itchy and look like small cauliflower-shaped flesh-colored lesions. There is no cure for HPV; treatment is aimed at removing the warts through freezing, application of acid, or the use of lasers. The immune system of the infected person is often able to keep the virus under control, and the person then has no further need for treatment. It is estimated that more than 50% of sexually active men and women acquire genital HPV infection at some point in their lives.

Syphilis

Syphilis is caused by the bacterium *Treponema pallidum*. It has several stages of progression that may overlap. The main symptom of the first stage of syphilis is a painless sore called a chancre at the site of infection that can last from 10 to 90 days. The second stage is characterized by a rash on the entire body, including the palms of the hands and soles of the feet. The latent (hidden) stage of syphilis begins when the second-stage symptoms disappear. Without treatment, the infection remains in the body and can progress to the late stage. The late stage of syphilis can cause severe damage to the internal organs and may eventually lead to a loss of mental functions and death. The infection can be cured at any stage with antibiotics.

Trichomoniasis

Trichomoniasis is a vaginal infection caused by *Trichomonas vaginalis*, a **protozoan**. Signs and symptoms of infection range from being asymptomatic to very symptomatic. Typical symptoms in women include a foul-smelling discharge from the vagina, burning with urination, and vaginal bleeding. Most men who get this infection do not experience symptoms. The disease is generally treated with the antibiotic metronidazole.

THE HISTORY OF GONORRHEA

Gonorrhea is not a new disease. It dates back further than most other sexually transmitted diseases. Ancient Chinese and Middle Eastern records dating to 3500 B.C. describe a disease resembling gonorrhea. Many classical Greek medical writings recognized the illness as a blockage of the urinary tract in males. The disease was most evident in males and was often confused with other diseases in females. For the most part, it was not readily identified (and often still is not) in many females.

One of the earliest descriptions of sexually transmitted diseases comes from Chinese Emperor Huang Ti in 2600 B.C. His medical manuscripts include a chapter that details information about STDs, including gonorrhea. The book of Leviticus, from the Old Testament of the Bible, contains an obvious description of gonorrhea with urethral discharge: "Any man hath a running issue out of his flesh, because of this issue he is unclean." The Greek physician Galen (Figure 2.3) (A.D. 130–200) is credited with naming gonorrhea from the Greek words *gonos* (meaning "semen") and *rhoia* ("to flow"). He likely mistakenly believed that the discharge that often occurs in men who have the disease was an involuntary loss of semen.

By the end of the 16th century, sexually transmitted diseases were recognized to be more common among prostitutes and

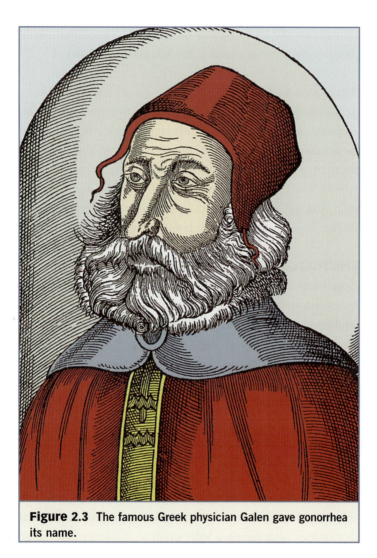

Figure 2.3 The famous Greek physician Galen gave gonorrhea its name.

people who were sexually promiscuous. The evolution of the word *clap* as a slang name for gonorrhea is derived from the small shelters in France known as *clapiers* (literally meaning "rabbit huts") where prostitutes often lived. At this time, men were seen as victims and women as the cause of STDs such as gonorrhea. The basic biology of the female reproductive system was mistakenly thought to breed diseases, since it was believed to provide a source of heat and moisture that helped germs grow. The condom has been advocated as a disease prevention method since the 1700s.

Outbreaks of STDs have been associated throughout history with wars. There is evidence that ancient Roman soldiers fighting with Julius Caesar (100–44 B.C.) had gonorrhea. During the Crimean War (A.D. 1854–1856), sexually transmitted diseases caused almost as many deaths as malnutrition, tuberculosis, and dysentery. By 1896, only 37% of the British troops occupying India had never had an STD. Nearly 60 years later, soldiers during World War II (1939–1945) were the first to receive large-scale education about STDs and their prevention. A significant part of this education, however, continued to reinforce the belief that women were the source of infection.

Communicable diseases of all types have also been spread by migration and trade throughout history. The spread of infections is attributed to traders (such as fur traders) and explorers. The medical reports of the Lewis and Clark expedition (1803–1806) include a description of expedition members acquiring gonorrhea from the Mandan Indians in North Dakota and the Chinook and Clatsop Indians of Oregon. These infections, however, probably originated from the crews of the fur trading ships that frequented these areas before Lewis and Clark arrived, not from the Indians themselves.

THE DISCOVERY OF THE GONORRHEA BACTERIUM

The search for the cause of gonorrhea took many turns throughout history as well. In the 18th century, the English physician Benjamin Bell believed that gonorrhea could result from anything that caused the urethra to become inflamed, including horseback riding and becoming overheated. Scientists at the time believed that a warm body not only received infection more readily but also enhanced transmission of the infection by making it more poisonous. They believed that body heat was intensified by wine, a spicy diet, and sexual excitement.

Early doctors spoke of all STDs as a single ailment. For example, they thought that syphilis and gonorrhea were the same disease, or that gonorrhea was the first stage of syphilis. The confusion about the two diseases remained until a large study of 2,500 patients conducted by Philippe Record in 1838

HISTORY OF THE CONDOM

A.D. 100–200 Scenes in cave paintings in France depict condoms.

1500s Italian anatomist Fallopius describes a sheath of linen used to protect men against syphilis; the first condoms with **spermicides** are made from linen sheaths soaked in chemical solution and allowed to dry prior to use.

1640 Condoms made of fish and animal intestines are used in England.

c. 1660–1685 A man named Dr. Condom invents a sheath to help British King Charles II avoid fathering illegitimate children.

1706 First published use of word *condum* appears in a poem.

1844 Condom manufacturing is revolutionized by the discovery of rubber vulcanization (which turns rubber into strong elastic material) by Goodyear.

1861 *The New York Times* publishes the first American condom advertisement.

1873 The Comstock law makes advertising birth control illegal and allows the postal service to confiscate condoms sent through the mail.

proved that syphilis and gonorrhea were not the same illness. It was not until the invention of the electron microscope in the 1930s that scientists acquired the ability to examine the bacteria that caused STDs such as gonorrhea and syphilis, and were able to identify them as separate entities.

1935 U.S. manufacturers produce 1.5 million condoms a day.

1942 Condoms are issued to soldiers during the landing at Dunkerque, France, to cover and protect rifle barrels from salt water.

1957 Durex makes the first lubricated condom in Great Britain.

1960s The availability of the birth control pill leads to a decrease in the use of condoms.

1977 The U.S. Supreme Court decides in *Carey* v. *Population Services* that a state may not prohibit minors from buying over-the-counter contraceptives.

1980s Condom use increases with the onset of the HIV/AIDS epidemic.

1990s Colored and flavored condoms appear on the market.

1992 The female condom is introduced.

1994 The first polyurethane condom is introduced for men.

The development of **germ theory**, which is attributed to French scientist Louis Pasteur (1822–1895) in the 1860s, paved the way for many changes in the science of **microbiology** (Figure 2.4). Germ theory defied conventional wisdom to state that **microorganisms** were present in the air but were not created *by* air; most scientists up until this time believed that organisms developed spontaneously. **Gram staining** (see Box on page 38) and culture systems (methods of growing samples of microorganisms) allowed bacteria to be identified in the laboratory. The bacterium responsible for gonorrhea (*Neisseria gonorrhoeae*) was named after Albert Neisser (1854–1916), a German scientist who first isolated the bacterium in 1879 (see Box on page 26).

EARLY TREATMENT OF GONORRHEA

Treatment of the disease has had a similarly long history. By the year A.D. 1200, more than 1,400 medications had been employed to treat gonorrhea, though most of them were not effective. Scientists performed experiments in the 1700s to try to find useful treatments for gonorrhea by infecting men with the pus from individuals who had the disease. These subjects then received the experimental treatment methods to evaluate the effect. The process of infecting otherwise healthy individuals with the goal of treating them experimentally would certainly be discouraged by the institutional review panels that exist today (see Box on page 27).

In the 18th century, the treatment of gonorrhea was based on the quantity and quality of pus from the urethra. People with mild symptoms were given bland fluids and various oral treatments, or simply left untreated. Severe symptoms resulted in more extreme treatments, including **bloodletting** and urethral lavage. Patients who agreed to try urethral lavage truly must have desired a cure. The painful process involved placing a catheter (tube) through the urethra of the penis, which was then flushed with 114–122°F (46–50°C) water in whatever

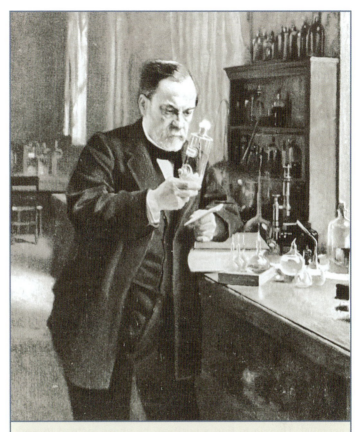

Figure 2.4 Louis Pasteur, pictured here in his laboratory, developed the germ theory in the 1860s. This new idea stated that microorganisms caused disease.

quantity the patient could tolerate. In the historical medical descriptions, the doctors report that the greater the patient's discomfort, the better the results. This treatment was repeated for two to three consecutive days; additional treatments were based on the continued presence of symptoms—and probably whether or not the patient chose to return!

Private doctors and some hospitals were reluctant to care for patients with sexually transmitted diseases in the early 20th century because those infected were considered immoral.

The social attitude of the time held that their promiscuous sexual behavior was the cause of the disease and, therefore, the patients did not deserve medical care. People infected with sexually transmitted diseases were forced to turn to lay practitioners and over-the-counter remedies. This likely resulted in the further spread of the disease, since these treatments did nothing to cure gonorrhea.

Hope for the treatment of gonorrhea grew with the discovery of the antibiotic penicillin in 1928 and its widespread use to kill bacterial infections during the 1940s.

ALBERT NEISSER, DISCOVERER OF THE GONORRHEA BACTERIUM

Albert Ludwig Sigesmund Neisser was born in Germany on January 22, 1855. His father was a well-known local physician in the town of Schweidnitz, where the family lived.

Neisser went to the nearby city of Breslau in 1872 to study medicine, as his father had done before him. Although he was not an outstanding student, he eventually passed his courses and went off to look for work as an internal medicine specialist. Unable to find a position, he chose instead to work in a dermatology clinic run by Dr. Oskar Simon. There, in 1879, when he was just 24 years old, Neisser discovered the bacterium that now bears his name—*Neisseria gonorrhoeae*. Figuring out what was causing the disease that had plagued humanity since recorded history began was no small achievement. However, even though the cause of gonorrhea was known, it was not until antibiotics were discovered in the early 20th century and brought into widespread use in the late 1930s and early 1940s that the disease could actually be cured. Still, Neisser has won a place in the history of medicine as the "father of gonococcus."

During World War II (the United States entered the war in 1941), the Army Navy Public Health Service and the National Research Council were able to pool their resources for medical investigations. This research, education, and treatment boom

ETHICAL REVIEW PANELS

Have you ever heard or seen an advertisement recruiting subjects for a research study about a new medication or treatments and wondered if you should be in the research study? What precautions are taken to make sure that scientists are testing new products safely?

The Food and Drug Administration (FDA) has established guidelines for Institutional Review Boards (IRB) to protect the rights of human subjects involved in scientific research. All research that involves human subjects must be reviewed by a group of people (doctors, nurses, social workers, clergy, psychologists, and people from the community) to ensure that human rights are not violated in the interest of science and discovery. The purpose of IRB review is to make sure, both before the research starts and periodically throughout the study, that all possible steps are taken to protect the rights and welfare of people participating as subjects in the research. The experiment or project is reviewed for potential harm to humans, to be certain that the research is not taking unfair advantage of subjects, and that the information the subjects receive before agreeing to take part is clear and complete. Research projects will be stopped by the IRB if any violations of human rights are found or if unexpected problems are discovered as the project progresses.

If you are considering participating in a research study, make sure the researcher clearly describes all the possible risks involved for you. Taking part in scientific research is an excellent way to learn about how science works in the everyday world.

was so effective in reducing the incidence of gonorrhea that it led to the misguided belief by the 1950s that gonorrhea had been completely eliminated as a health threat. Federal funding for gonorrhea research stopped, forcing the closing of STD clinics and medical school departments. Condom distribution programs that had been started in the 1940s essentially disappeared. Compounding the effect of this change in public policy, after the development of the birth control pill in the 1960s, the use of barrier contraceptive devices such as condoms declined significantly. These factors resulted in the rate of gonorrhea increasing by 250% between 1966 and 1976. The number of cases of gonorrhea began to decline in the mid-1980s and continued to decline through the 1990s, mainly because of the advent of the HIV/AIDS epidemic, which scared many people into returning to the use of condoms. As we will see in Chapter 6, recent data shows that this trend is now reversing itself, particularly among teens—a dangerous development that has caused great concern among health-care professionals.

In the next chapter, we will take a look at the bacterium that causes gonorrhea in close detail, and see how it gets into the body and leads to infection.

3

What Is Gonorrhea and How Does It Affect the Body?

What living things can claim the following?

- Outnumber human cells in our body

- Can ward off infection

- Help facilitate digestion

- Are used in the production of wine, cheese, and yogurt

- Help compost our trash.

Do you give up? The answer is bacteria. Bacteria can do all these things and more. Although they have a reputation for causing serious disease and illness, bacteria are underappreciated for the many positive things they bring to our everyday lives. In fact, the majority of bacteria are harmless to humans and many are actually helpful to us. The bacterium that causes gonorrhea, however, as we will see, is not one of the majority.

CHARACTERISTICS OF BACTERIA

Bacteria and viruses came into existence long before human beings. Human evolution basically provided a new group of hosts for the growth of bacteria and viruses. A **host** is an organism that another organism uses as a place to live and obtain the food and nutrients it needs to survive.

Today, bacteria and viruses cause most human infections throughout the world. Bacteria and viruses are called **microbes**, or tiny organisms too small to be seen without a microscope. Many people are familiar with the terms *bacterium* and *virus* but do not actually understand the difference between the two types of microbes. The first way to tell bacteria and viruses apart is by size. Viruses are significantly smaller than bacteria. The largest viruses are equal in size to the smallest bacteria. An average-sized virus is between 20 and 250 nanometers (a nanometer is equal to one-billionth of a meter). The average bacteria are about 4 times larger, or 1,000 nanometers. Bacteria are single-celled living organisms and are more complicated in structure than viruses. (There is actually some controversy among medical professionals over whether viruses are even living things at all, since they depend entirely on their host to survive and multiply.) Bacteria usually have rigid cell walls and a thin surface membrane that surrounds the fluid inside the cell, called the **cytoplasm**. In contrast, a virus is very simple: It has a protein coat and a core of genetic material. It may or may not have an outer spiky layer called an envelope.

Bacteria are able to reproduce on their own because they contain all the genetic information they need to copy themselves. They can live in nearly every environment, including water, ice, soil, plants, and animals. Viruses, on the other hand, do not contain the structures they need to reproduce. To multiply, they must invade a host cell and take over its functions, forcing it to make copies of the virus instead of performing its usual job. When outside of a living cell, a virus is **dormant**, or inactive.

COMMENSAL BACTERIA

Neisseria gonorrhoeae, the microbe that causes gonorrhea, comes from a family of bacteria that normally live commensally on many animals. **Commensal** organisms gain benefits from another organism without harming their host. Commensals exist because of a long relationship with the host. People often forget about these bacteria because they generally cause no health problems. The human body is host to many commensal bacteria. They are invisibly spread throughout the body. Most of these bacteria are found in the digestive system and help us process the food we eat. However, many live contentedly on the mucous membranes and skin. Commensal bacteria usually feed on nutrients found in human secretions such as mucus and sweat. (Mucus is a gummy material composed of carbohydrates partly edible to the bacteria. It is rich in amino acids, minerals, and sugars that are beneficial for bacterial growth. Its high water content provides a moist growing environment.) Mucous membranes are found in the digestive system, respiratory system, and genitourinary tract.

The mucous membranes of the lower digestive system are an even better environment for commensals. They are loaded with plenty of food that has already been broken down by host **enzymes** into readily available nutrients. Many commensals feed on material that cannot be digested by the host, which means that there is no competition for food between the commensal and the host—one reason the commensal is not harmful. Almost all the commensal bacteria live in the large intestine. It is a stable environment full of food. The stomach and small intestine are harsh environments for many bacteria. Only a few bacteria can live in the caustic, acidic environment of the stomach. Most bacteria are digested here or their chemistry is disrupted to the point where they cannot survive. One exception is the notorious bacterium *Helicobacter pylori*, which lives comfortably in the stomach and upper part of the small intestine. These bacteria have been proven to cause stomach ulcers—sores that form in the stomach and become further irritated by stomach acids.

Skin is a rich source of food for many microbes. However, it is exposed to any environmental conditions encountered by the host. Only the subtle warmth of the blood underneath the skin and the moisture of sweat provide microbes any protection. Skin commensals feed mainly on the nutrient-rich sweat and oils. Like mucus, sweat contains amino acids, minerals, and sugars. Skin oils provide a good source of fat that is helpful for the energy needs of microbes trying to survive the unforgiving conditions of the skin. Some microbes such as fungi eat the outer layer of dead skin cells, called the stratum squamosum. The continuous shedding of the stratum squamosum poses a problem for skin bacteria. They end up being removed from the skin as the stratum squamosum cells flake off. Cast-off stratum squamosum cells from the scalp are commonly called dandruff. To avoid falling off, many of these bacteria try to live around the openings of glands, where they are less likely to be removed.

Some commensals do provide a small benefit to the host by keeping harmful bacteria out of the body. They do this by competing for food and space. Sometimes they also produce secretions that inhibit the growth of other microbes. Several of these secretions are now being investigated by scientists to help develop specific treatments for microbial infections. Bacteria in the female genitourinary tract act in this manner to keep down the growth of the vaginal yeast *Candida albicans*. The yeast reciprocates by hindering the growth of the bacteria. In this way, a balance is achieved, and neither organism is able to multiply out of control. This interaction—when a noticeable benefit occurs between the microbe and the host—is called mutualism. In many situations, it is very difficult to tell the difference between commensalism and mutualism. The benefits provided by microbes are not always obvious until the microbes are eliminated from the body. Long-term antibiotic treatments give evidence of this. The antibiotics often wipe out commensals, resulting in a variety of ill effects. For example, certain antibiotics destroy the bacteria that keep yeast under control in the female genitourinary tract, and women frequently come down with yeast infections as a result of the loss of these beneficial bacteria.

Commensals are good for the body as long as their numbers are kept in control and they remain in the body regions where they normally reside. The body's immune system is the main factor that keeps commensalism and mutualism in check. Microbes are regularly culled by the immune system components of the mucous membranes and the skin. Mucous membranes have chemical and physical barriers that keep microbes from entering the body and unintentionally causing disease. Chemical barriers somehow kill or impede the growth of the microbes. The acidic environment of the stomach prevents the growth of most microbes, especially bacteria. Immune system cells called white blood cells produce certain chemical barriers. These white blood cells produce secretions that kill microbes or help with their removal. Physical barriers literally block the microbes from entering particular body regions. The tight connections attaching digestive system cells and skin cells act as barricades that keep bacteria on the surface.

WHEN GOOD BACTERIA GO BAD

Harmless bacteria can become pathogenic (disease-causing) if they acquire genetic changes that alter their survival characteristics. Certain types of genetic changes are called mutations. Mutations are usually caused by mistakes made during cell division that "rewrite" the organism's genetic information. Sometimes mutations can lead bacteria to produce unique secretions that can harm the host. Mutations can change the dietary needs of bacteria, forcing them to compete with the host for nutrition. They can also throw off the delicate interactions between different commensals. Mutations occur naturally as bacteria reproduce. Chemicals called mutagens can also cause them. Mutagens include certain types of petroleum-based chemicals and pesticides. The ultraviolet (UV) light that leads to sunburns and radiation poisoning are other causes of mutation. Another way for bacteria to make genetic changes is through sexual reproduction. Many bacteria pick up small

(continued on page 36)

THE HUMAN IMMUNE SYSTEM

The human body has a very complicated and well-coordinated set of techniques to help protect us against disease. The organs and cells that carry out these self-protection techniques are collectively called the immune system (Figure 3.1).

The body's first line of defense is made up of physical barriers that help stop pathogens (like bacteria) from getting inside the cells. The largest of these barriers is the skin. We also have other barriers, including mucous membranes (which can trap pathogens in sticky mucus and help the body expel them through coughing, sneezing, or in some cases, urination and defecation), and cilia (hair-like structures in the nose, lungs, and other organs that help sweep foreign substances out of the body). Before it can start a successful infection, the disease-causing microorganism has to find a way past these physical defenses. This often occurs through cuts or open wounds on the skin, which allow the pathogen direct access to the bloodstream.

Once the pathogen gets inside the body, the immune system responds with a second line of defense. The immune system has many different kinds of cells, all of which play very special roles in destroying invaders and helping the body repair any damage that might be done by invading organisms. Among the immune cells that attack the invader first are macrophages—large cells that literally gobble up invading organisms and kill them. (*Macro* refers to the large part of a cell, while *phage* means "eater of.")

Macrophages cannot eliminate a pathogen entirely on their own, however. To continue the attack on the invader, the immune system also has white blood cells, or lymphocytes (also called B cells and T cells), that help stop an infection.

B cells are found in the blood, where they are constantly traveling, searching for foreign organisms that may have entered the body. When they find cells or particles they do not recognize

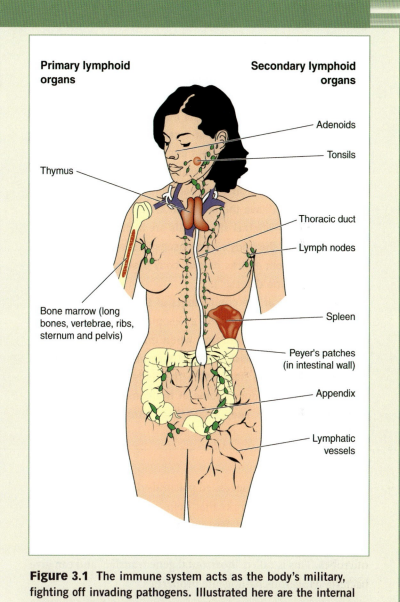

Figure 3.1 The immune system acts as the body's military, fighting off invading pathogens. Illustrated here are the internal immune system organs (the body's second line of defense). These organs help eliminate harmful pathogens if they have breached the first line of defense (skin and mucous membranes).

(known as antigens), they attach to them and produce anti-bodies—proteins that will remain in the body even after the infection is over to help the immune system recognize a particular pathogen quickly if it ever enters the body again.

Meanwhile, T cells also play a major role in the immune response. There are two types of T cells. Helper T cells locate invading pathogens and send out chemical signals to the rest of the body to let the immune system know an invader has entered. Killer T cells, on the other hand, not only recognize invaders, but also have the ability to attach to and destroy unfamiliar cells—whether these cells are bacteria, viruses, or even the cells of the body's own tissues in some cases (when the immune system attacks its own body tissues, this is referred to as "autoimmune disease").

Together, all of the components of the human immune system are generally very good at keeping the body healthy, but they can be outnumbered when enough bacteria or other pathogens get inside body cells and begin to multiply, causing an infection. It is often the body's own response to infection that produces some of the common signs and symptoms of disease, such as swelling, fever, and the creation of pus.

(continued from page 33)

pieces of genetic material called plasmids during reproduction. Plasmids carry many traits that help the bacteria get past the body's immune system defenses. Certain bacteria pick up small chunks of genetic material from decaying organisms and dead microbes. This is called "horizontal gene transfer" and can give bacteria dangerous pathogenic properties.

THE *NEISSERIA GONORRHOEAE* BACTERIUM

Neisseria gonorrhoeae (Figure 3.2), the organism that causes gonorrhea, is a gram-negative bacterium that only infects

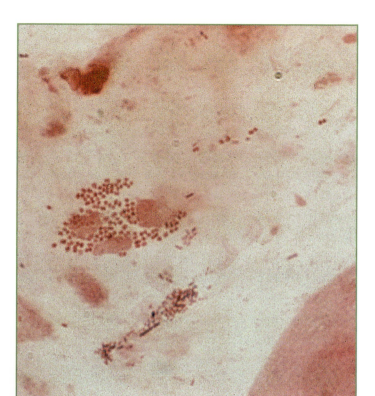

Figure 3.2 *Neisseria gonorrhoeae* (seen here as small pink dots) is a small, spherical, gram-negative bacterium. Gram-negative organisms stain pink when subjected to the Gram stain procedure, because of the the way their cell walls are structured.

humans (see the Box on page 38 for an explanation of Gram stains and how bacteria are classified with this method). It is probably derived from *Neisseria meningitidis* (a bacterium that infects the lining of the brain and spinal cord), but has learned to live instead on the mucous membranes of the genitourinary tract. Transmission of the bacterium occurs from human to human, primarily through sexual conduct; once outside the body of the human host, the bacterium cannot survive for long. This is why it is very difficult, if not impossible (contrary to popular belief), to catch gonorrhea from inanimate objects such as toilet seats.

The *Neisseria gonorrhoeae* bacterium is very successful as a pathogen because it is able to defend against the human

THE GRAM STAIN TEST

The Gram stain test is an important technique for bacteriologists and clinicians. The process itself has changed little since Hans Christian Gram originally developed it in 1884. Hans Christian Gram, a Danish doctor working in Berlin, accidentally stumbled upon a method that now forms the basis for identifying bacteria. While examining diseased lung tissue, he discovered that certain stains were taken up and retained by the bacterial cells. He developed a staining procedure that divided nearly all types of bacteria into two groups—gram-negative and gram-positive.

The purpose of the technique is to differentiate between two groups of bacteria based on their cell wall structure. The first step in the Gram stain process is to "heat fix" a sample of cells to a slide by passing it several times through a flame. The cells are then stained with crystal violet, a basic dye that is absorbed by all bacteria in equal quantities. In the third step, the cells are fixed to the slide with an iodine solution and washed briefly with alcohol to remove the stain. The final step is the application of a lighter-colored dye (safranin) to "counterstain" the cell. When observed under a microscope, gram-positive organisms maintain the original violet coloring, while gram-negative bacteria lose the violet color and show the pink counterstain instead. This difference in staining reflects a fundamental difference in the way the bacterial cell wall is structured (see Table 3.1). Gram-positive bacteria have body's attempts to eliminate it and is able to survive in the host without causing significant damage—at least at first. Scientists who studied gonorrhea in the 1960s were astounded to observe that *Neisseria gonorrhoeae* can sometimes remain in the body

a relatively thick wall that is composed of many layers of a substance called peptidoglycan. Gram-negative bacteria (like *Neisseria gonorrhoeae*) have only a thin layer of peptidoglycan, surrounded by a thin outer membrane made of lipopolysaccharide, or endotoxin. Many species of gram-negative bacteria can cause disease. This capability is usually associated with the endotoxin component of their cell wall.

Table 3.1 Gram-negative Versus Gram-positive Bacteria

Gram-negative Bacteria	Gram-positive Bacteria
• Appear pink on gram stain	• Appear purple on gram stain
• Double membrane around each bacterial cell	• Broad, dense single cell wall
• Cell wall rich in lipopoly-saccharide provides permeability barrier	• Cell wall rich in peptidoglycan provides strength and rigidity
• Protective outer membrane increases resistance to peni-cillin (a common antibiotic)	• More sensitive to (more easily killed by) penicillin
• Contains endotoxin	• Does not contain endotoxin

without harming the infected person at all. The bacterium causes an immune response. A sure indication of gonorrhea is the inflammation of the infected tissues followed by the formation of pus. Pus is produced as the body mounts an attack against invading microbes. The pus produced in the penis is readily seen and is what gave gonorrhea the slang name "drip." Another ignoble name for gonorrhea was "racehorse," which refers to the way the pus in the male continuously runs out of the end of the urethra. In spite of inducing inflammation and the production of pus, *Neisseria gonorrhoeae* somehow evades many of the defenses of the immune system. Current research now shows that *Neisseria gonorrhoeae* is capable of blocking some of the activities of white blood cells called macrophages. Macrophages digest invading organisms during an infection. Digestion by macrophages is called phagocytosis. The same structure (called a "pilus;" the plural form is *pili*) that permits *Neisseria gonorrhoeae* to attach to cells also inhibits macrophage phagocytosis. By doing this, the bacterium reduces the ability of the immune system to fight off *Neisseria gonorrhoeae* and other disease organisms. This makes it common for people with gonorrhea to be easily infected with other sexually transmitted diseases.

How does inhibiting phagocytosis permit disease organisms to remain in the body unaffected by the immune system? Macrophage phagocytosis is the first step in determining if microbes or foreign matter are invading the body. Upon finding a microbe, the macrophage kills and digests the organism. It then changes its cell membrane in a way that tells the immune system about the invading microbe. It labels itself with proteins (called **antigens**) found on the surface of the microbe. The proteins then act as a signal, telling other immune system cells about what kind of microbe has entered the body. Lymphocytes (white blood cells) called B cells use this information to produce protective proteins called **antibodies**.

Antibodies stick to the microbe, with various outcomes. One outcome is that the antibodies prevent *Neisseria gonorrhoeae* and other microbes from sticking to body cells. Another effect of antibodies is that they label the microbes for destruction by macrophages and other white blood cells. Another group of white blood cells, called T cells, also use the signal sent out by macrophages to enhance the immune response. Helper T cells produce a variety of secretions that stimulate the immune system, while cytotoxic, or killer, T cells produce poisons that kill the invading microbes.

STRUCTURE OF *NEISSERIA GONORRHOEAE*

The surface components of the gonorrhea bacterium are typical of a gram-negative bacterium. The surface structures include pili (hair-like appendages on the surface of the cell; see Figure 3.3); opa, or outer membrane proteins (which work as a sort of glue to hold the bacteria to the cell wall); and lipo-oligosaccharide (LOS), a surface substance that is thought to be responsible for many of the symptoms of gonorrhea. These components direct the bacterium's interaction with the host cell, including how the bacterium attaches to the cell and invades the outer lining of the host cell. Infection occurs when the pili affix themselves to the outer lining of the host cell membrane (called the **epithelium**). Genetic variability may occur at any one of these three surface components of the bacteria. Therefore, the human immune system is not always able to recognize and eliminate the infecting organism.

GONORRHEA BACTERIA IN THE BODY

Neisseria gonorrhoeae can enter the bloodstream in both females and males through sores on the mucous membranes. In the blood, they can damage the heart, joints, kidneys, and liver. *Neisseria gonorrhoeae* normally enters the body through the mucous membranes of the genitourinary system. In males, it enters the body through the small opening near the end of

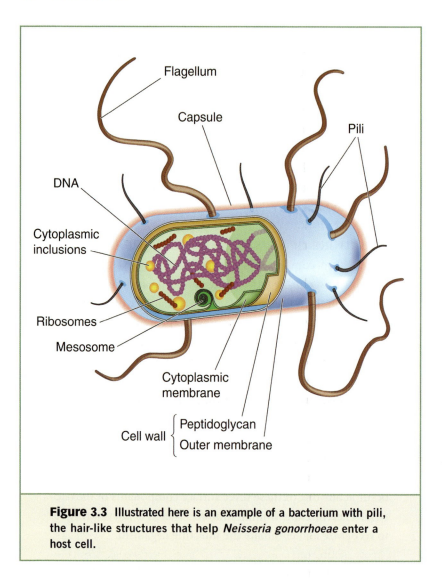

Figure 3.3 Illustrated here is an example of a bacterium with pili, the hair-like structures that help *Neisseria gonorrhoeae* enter a host cell.

the urethra. *Neisseria gonorrhoeae* usually makes first contact with the female body at the upper region of the vagina. Other **portals of entry** (places where a microbe enters the body) for *Neisseria gonorrhoeae* include the eyes, rectum, and throat. *Neisseria gonorrhoeae* does not require any special features to make contact with the portal of entry. It does not have to enter the blood, like its relative *Neisseria meningitidis*, which causes meningococcal meningitis (an inflammation of the meninges, the tissues that surround the brain and spinal cord). Gonorrhea affects the surface of the mucous membranes. As a result, it does not need the enzymes and toxins (poisons) other bacteria need to penetrate body surfaces. *Neisseria meningitidis*, for example, can only cause disease by using enzymes and toxins that break down body tissues, allowing entry into the bloodstream.

Once the bacteria get into the body, the human immune system produces cytokines that cause inflammation to fight the infection. **Cytokines** are small proteins that help regulate immunity. They are only produced in response to a foreign substance that gets inside the body and stimulates the immune system. Many cells such as lymphocytes, phagocytes, and epithelial (on the surface, such as the skin or the lining of body organs) cells produce cytokines in response to different stimuli such as trauma, blood loss, tumors, viruses, and bacteria. The interaction between the gonorrhea bacteria and the cytokines produces an intense inflammatory reaction that leads to a **purulent**, or pus-like, discharge that oozes from the membranes. The gonorrhea bacteria are present in this discharge, which allows for the diagnosis of gonorrhea from samples of these secretions. In males, the pus continuously runs out of the end of the urethra. The pus is not always visible in females and is usually first detected by a health-care provider's examination—not noticed by the patient herself. Further irritation can cause scarring to the infected tissue, bringing about more pain and the chance of contracting other infections. It is possible for the bacteria to move up the reproductive tract, causing infertility in both females and males. In females, the bacteria can pass into the abdominal cavity, causing pelvic inflammatory disease (PID). This potentially fatal condition damages the reproductive organs and can spread to the blood, sometimes leading to death.

The gonorrhea bacterium theoretically should have limited capability to survive because it has only one possible host:

humans. The bacterium, however, has survived for thousands of years because of its antigenic variability—its ability to produce many different kinds of antigens, which makes the body's immunity to one type of antigen unable to protect against another. The bacterium is able to change both its **phenotype**, or its observable characteristics, and its **genotype**, or specific genetic makeup. Phenotypic variability occurs through constantly changing the appearance of the genome by turning parts of it off and on. Think of this as having a combination lock and constantly changing the combination to outwit the immune system's attempt to open the lock. Genotypic variability is achieved through two processes: The bacterium either takes on new genetic material, or mutates (changes) the genetic material it already has.

The battle between the infected person and the bacteria is thus best described as a continual arms race. The bacteria responds to the host's immune system defenses by changing its genetic components, which results in a further response from the immune system of the host, which starts the whole process over again.

HOW *NEISSERIA GONORRHOEAE* CAUSES DISEASE

Pathogenesis means the ability to cause disease. The survival of a communicable disease in the body unfortunately causes some degree of illness, or pathology. Under most conditions, commensal organisms are able to live in or on the body with no ill effect. But many organisms, or pathogens, produce diseases that are barely detectable by a health-care provider or noticeable by the host. Parasitic worms such as pinworm can live for years in the intestine. The biggest problem they cause is mild irritation of the anus and nostrils.

Extremely harmful pathogens cause diseases such as AIDS and syphilis. Both of these STDs produce ailments that can lead to premature death. AIDS is obviously the most ruthless of the STDs because it usually results in the failure of the body to fight disease, and eventually kills the victim (although it can take many years before the first symptoms appear). Syphilis, too, can take many years to slowly kill a person. Influenza is the ultimate rapid-onset pathogen, having the ability to cause death within just a few days of acquiring the virus. Like gonorrhea, influenza does most of its damage at the portal of entry. Influenza's portal of the entry is the lining of the lungs.

Neisseria gonorrhoeae has a highly variable pathology, ranging from undetectably mild to noticeably destructive and painful. Unfortunately, it is difficult to predict how any individual person would respond to an infection with *Neisseria gonorrhoeae.*

Bacterial pathology is based on a combination of the portal of entry and the cell wall characteristics of the particular bacterium. (Antibiotics kill bacteria by interfering with the cell wall, so the type of cell wall dictates which types of antibiotics will effectively kill a certain bacterium.) Bacteria that live in the blood and internal organs initially create problems as they erode tissues to make their way into the body. The damage caused by getting inside the body produces an ailment in itself. But it also leaves the body vulnerable to other organisms, producing a condition called "secondary disease." Secondary diseases are sometimes called "complications." Many secondary diseases are caused by normally harmless commensals that enter parts of the body where they do not belong. They then unintentionally damage whatever body part they have invaded. Vaginal yeast may cause fatal secondary infections if it enters the blood and makes its way to the brain. Mutualistic intestinal bacteria will also produce disease—including life-threatening nervous system conditions and kidney damage—by invading through sores produced by pathogens in the digestive system. *Neisseria gonorrhoeae* causes the types of irritation that permit secondary infections.

As mentioned, cell wall characteristics play a predictable role in pathology. Gram-negative bacteria such as *Neisseria gonorrhoeae* release potent poisons called endotoxins. Endotoxins are released by the cell wall during bacterial death and reproduction. These toxins are some of the most potent cell-killing substances known. They are critically monitored by health officials to ensure that they do not end up in prepared foods, medications, and drinking water. Even small amounts of endotoxins cause severe cell damage, resulting in the complete failure of many body organs. The cell walls of gram-positive bacteria, on the other hand, produce no ill effects to the host. To an extent, they harm the host by secreting a broad group of chemicals called exotoxins, which have many specific effects on the body. Cell damage, fever, kidney failure, and rashes are all signs of exotoxins. Some people are allergic to exotoxins, which further complicates the pathology. Others perceive extreme pain when exotoxins are present in the blood or are in contact with a particular tissue.

The degree of pathology also depends on the host's immune system. More and more people with gonorrhea also have other communicable diseases, both because their lifestyle (most infected people have multiple sexual partners and engage in unprotected intercourse) and previous infection with gonorrhea makes them vulnerable to other infections that are acquired in the same way (through sexual activity). In some cases, it is beneficial to have one disease precede another because this activates the immune system. However, the presence of two debilitating diseases may put too much strain on the immune system. One disease can go relatively untouched as the immune system concentrates on battling the other ailment. Millions of people in many developing nations carry large amounts of parasitic protozoans and worms in their bodies throughout much of their lives. This chronic, or long-term, condition reduces the body's ability to fight off microbes. Gonorrhea thrives when the immune system is not working up to its full capacity. Thus, people who have it are more likely to contract sexually transmitted diseases upon immediate contact, whereas healthy people are more likely to be able to fight off the bacteria if the initial infection is small.

HOW GONORRHEA IS SPREAD

Communicable diseases rely on the fact that they can exit the body to infect another person. The means by which a microbe leaves the body is called the portal of exit. There are a variety of ways that microbes can leave the body. Sneezing releases cold and influenza viruses from the respiratory system of an infected person. The viruses are carried to the next person in the sprayed-out mucus and saliva, or droplets. Many organisms that invade the respiratory system use this portal of exit. Gonorrhea, being an STD, is transferred almost exclusively from host to host by unprotected sexual contact. The bacterium travels in the mucus released by the penis or the vagina. Gonorrhea is more readily transferred from males to females, because the female body has a much larger surface area of mucous membrane the bacteria can penetrate. Males contract gonorrhea about 30–50% of the time during intercourse with an infected person. Infected males pass along gonorrhea to females with a 60–90% chance of infection.

Other types of contact with infected mucus can occasionally spread gonorrhea between individuals. For example, gonorrhea has been shown to transfer from one person to another when the people share undergarments that are freshly soiled with infected mucus and urine.

Sometimes it is very difficult for a pathogen to exit the body. This is true for microbes that live in the blood and deep in body tissues. Many pathogens are carried out of the body by **vectors**. Vectors are organisms or objects that carry disease from one host to another. Organisms are usually called "biological vectors" and objects are called "mechanical vectors." Biting animals can serve as biological vectors for diseases carried in the blood. Saliva transferred by the bite of the animal into another animal or person's blood can carry microbes that are then inserted into the new host. This method of disease transmission has limitations. First, large amounts of the microbe must be present in the fluid being transferred. Second, the microbe must be able to survive for a period of time in the biological vector. It is very unlikely that gonorrhea is spread this way, even if *Neisseria gonorrhoeae* manages to get into the bloodstream through a bite or cut. Rumors have at times abounded about AIDS and other STDs being spread by mosquitoes. However, this is extremely improbable and has never been confirmed by epidemiologists (people who study diseases and how they spread).

Clothing, eating utensils, and unclean medical equipment are common mechanical vectors. Improperly sterilized needles used for illegal drug use and tattooing transfer various microbes that live on the skin and in the blood. As mentioned above, gonorrhea can be carried from one person to another on objects that contain contaminated mucus. Luckily, however, *Neisseria gonorrhoeae* does not survive for a long time outside of the body. It dies within minutes to hours on mechanical vectors. This means it is virtually impossible to contract gonorrhea by touching chairs, doorknobs, and toilet seats. It is also very unlikely that the microbe would survive in swimming pools. It is important to understand the way *Neisseria gonorrhoeae* does and does not spread, so you can ignore the rumors and focus on effective ways to protect yourself from the pathogen.

4

Symptoms and Diagnosis

Sixteen-year-old Marie has been suffering from fever, headache, malaise, and muscle aches for six days. Her mother becomes worried and decides to take Marie to the emergency room. At the hospital, Marie shows the doctor treating her a painful swelling on her left wrist that developed quickly that same morning. The doctor notices that Marie also has several lesions, or sores, near the swollen wrist, and similar lesions near both armpits. The sores appear to be necrotic, which means they are made of dying tissue. Marie's body temperature is 100°F (38°C), slightly above the normal body temperature of 98.6°F (37°C). However, she shows no other signs of disease on her genitals, ears, eyes, nose, or throat.

The doctor realizes that Marie is showing signs of what is called **disseminated gonorrhea**, a type of gonorrhea that spreads beyond the genitals to other parts of the body and is often confused with syphilis and other pathogenic bacterial diseases of the blood. Skin lesions like Marie's are characteristic of this form of gonorrhea (Figure 4.1).

The doctor asks Marie a series of questions to try confirm the initial diagnosis: Have you engaged in sexual activity? When was the last time you had sex? How well did you know your partner? Did you use a condom? Have you had any problems urinating or passing wastes? Reluctantly, Marie admits that she had sex with a guy she met at a party about a month ago and says that, although he used a condom, it broke during intercourse. She also says that she has noticed some minor burning while urinating over the past week or two.

The doctor immediately orders tests for gonorrhea, which include a genitourinary swab, a sample of fluid from the affected joint (Marie's wrist), and a blood test to evaluate Marie's immune system. The test results

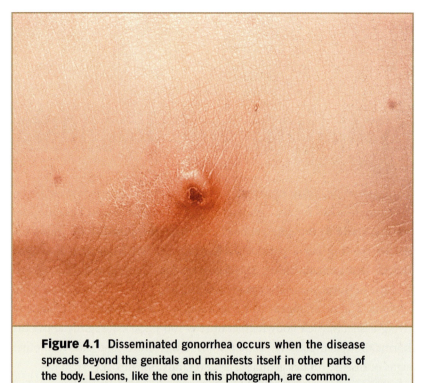

Figure 4.1 Disseminated gonorrhea occurs when the disease spreads beyond the genitals and manifests itself in other parts of the body. Lesions, like the one in this photograph, are common.

confirm that Marie does, indeed, have gonorrhea. She is relieved to learn that it is treatable, and the doctor admits her to the hospital to start a course of antibiotics under supervised care.

SYMPTOMS OF GONORRHEA

In Marie's case, the symptoms of her disease were obvious and made her uncomfortable enough to go to the hospital for help. Her case may be the exception to the rule, especially for women.

The early symptoms of gonorrhea are often mild, and some people who are infected have no symptoms of the disease; this is one reason why it is so readily transmitted. If they do show up, symptoms of gonorrhea usually appear anywhere from 2 to 57 days after sexual contact with an infected partner, with the average time being about 8 days. A small percentage of patients may be infected for several months without showing any symptoms.

The most typical symptoms of gonorrhea include painful urination, testicular or abdominal pain, and vaginal or penile discharge. This last symptom, the pus-like discharge, is what gave gonorrhea its slang name "the drip." This discharge is a result of the inflammation of the mucous membranes or lining of the urethra.

Although these are the most common symptoms of gonorrhea, the impact of the disease can vary widely, as you saw in Marie's case. Gonorrhea can range from an invasion of the host that produces no symptoms to a widespread infection that affects the joints, skin, heart, liver, and even the central nervous system (brain and spinal cord). How gonorrhea will affect a particular person is hard to predict. The number of bacteria found in an infected host does not necessarily indicate how severe the infection will be or how quickly it will develop. Asymptomatic gonorrhea infections are more common in teens, with 67% of males and 77% of females experiencing no symptoms. (Again, Marie was very lucky to have obvious symptoms that helped her discover her condition early enough to prevent severe damage to her body.) In contrast, the reported rate of asymptomatic infections among adults is 10% for men and 50% for women. These "hidden" infections may be due to the type of *Neisseria gonorrhoeae* that the host is carrying. Even small differences in the cell membrane proteins of *Neisseria gonorrhoeae* can affect how the bacteria spread and cause disease. In addition, the proteins are responsible for the strength of the body's immune response. You should recall that the gonorrhea bacterium comes from a family of commensal bacteria that often live harmlessly inside the human body. So, it is not unusual for some strains of *Neisseria gonorrhoeae* to be mild enough to live somewhat cooperatively within the body.

Sometimes the infection can be severe, however. Often, this occurs when the infected person has a hypersensitive (overly active) immune system. At least 1% of the population has a hypersensitivity called an allergy. Allergies result when the immune system overreacts to certain substances, such as pollen or mold. People with allergies are very likely to experience extreme immune reactions if they acquire *Neisseria gonorrhoeae*. This, in turn, makes the symptoms more severe because of the exaggerated irritation of body tissues and extra pus formation. It is also likely that people with this problem will come down with other infections because of the damage the gonorrhea causes. Other people, such as the elderly and infants, have slightly weakened immune systems that are not fully able to fight off disease. In these people, it is common for *Neisseria gonorrhoeae* to spread readily throughout the body.

Gonorrhea can result in infections of the genitals, **rectum**, throat, and eyes. Gonorrhea in the genitals of males will cause **urethritis** (inflammation of the urethra). Nearly half of all men who get gonorrhea will have discharge from the urethra. The second most common symptom is **dysuria**, or burning during urination. These symptoms may be transient and mild, and may go away without any treatment. Gonorrhea is one of many diseases that produce tiredness as the immune system attempts to fight off the infection. Malaise, like tiredness, occurs when the body is damaged and fighting disease. The term is best defined as a general feeling of being ill. Advanced cases of gonorrhea produce malaise. But again, many people feel well even though they may have been carrying around *Neisseria gonorrhoeae* for years.

When a woman has a gonorrhea infection, she usually will not have symptoms. If symptoms do exist, they normally consist of a **mucopurulent** (made up of mucus and pus) discharge from the vagina. Other nonspecific symptoms of gonorrhea include lower abdominal pain, bleeding, or pain during sexual intercourse. Changes in the menstrual period, such as spotting (bleeding between the normal periods) or increased bleeding with menstruation, may also result from a gonorrhea infection.

Gonorrhea in the rectum usually results from receptive anal intercourse with an infected partner. However, it has been reported in women who deny ever having anal intercourse. Scientists assume that these cases occurred when the **perineum** and **anus** were contaminated by **cervical secretions** after the woman had been previously infected with gonorrhea through vaginal intercourse. Rectal infection is usually confined to the lower 8 centimeters (cm) (3 inches) of the rectum and is often asymptomatic. The infected person may experience bloody or mucopurulent discharge from the anus, painful defecation, and occasionally diarrhea. Rectal gonorrhea is more difficult to treat than cases that affect the genitals or other parts of the body because the normal bacteria of the rectum contain enzymes that can inactivate antibiotics.

FORMS OF GONORRHEA INFECTION
Gonoccocal Pharyngitis
A gonorrhea infection in the throat is referred to as **gonoccocal pharyngitis** and results in redness and swelling that may be accompanied by small pustules (blisters) on the tonsils and uvula. This may be the sole site of infection when oral-genital contact is the only sexual exposure to the gonorrhea bacterium. Unlike the throat, the mucous membranes of the mouth are usually able to resist infection from gonorrhea.

Gonococcal Ophthalmitis
In an adult, infection of the eye with gonorrhea (**gonococcal ophthalmitis**, Figure 4.2) usually occurs when someone touches his or her eye with a finger or hand that has been contaminated with bacteria-containing discharge from another part of the body. The infection causes eye irritation with a purulent discharge. In infants, gonoccocal ophthalmitis can be acquired as the newborn passes through the infected mother's birth canal. An infant with gonoccocal ophthalmitis will develop red eyes with a discharge that is watery at first but may

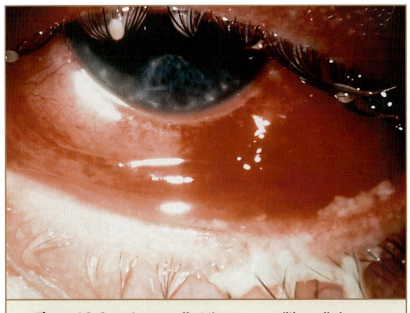

Figure 4.2 Gonorrhea can affect the eye, a condition called gono-coccal ophthalmitis. The eye may become red and have a purulent or bloody discharge. If left untreated, it can cause blindness.

become bloody within 3 days after birth. Infection in the eye may damage the cornea if not treated promptly, resulting in blindness. At the turn of the 19th century, nearly 25% of all blindness in the United States was caused by gonococcal ophthalmitis. The widespread treatment of all newborn infants with silver nitrate or erythromycin (an antibiotic) eyedrops in the delivery room has prevented gonococcal ophthalmitis and its complications by killing any gonorrhea bacteria the baby may have acquired during the birthing process.

DIAGNOSIS OF GONORRHEA

Early detection of gonorrhea is the key to preventing both the further spread of the disease and possibly dangerous complica-tions. Identification of gonorrhea is largely dependent upon evaluation as part of a routine health exam and the testing of people who are showing signs of the disease. Unfortunately, many infected people do not seek routine health checkups or are not offered sexually transmitted disease (STD) testing as part of a doctor's visit, especially if they are not experiencing symptoms. Even so, a diagnosis of gonorrhea can be made through a thorough examination of a patient.

The overall observation reviews any warning signs of disease that are easily visible to the health-care provider. This is a very critical step that requires special medical training and experience. Basically, the nurse, physician, or physician's assistant looks at various body regions for signs of disease. A sign is any measurable or visible indication that something is not normal. (A symptom, on the other hand, is something the patient reports, such as a headache.) Most of the signs of an STD are not very obvious upon a cursory inspection. In many cases, a person might have just recently picked up a communicable disease and has not yet begun to show any signs of infection. Gonorrhea has few obvious signs. This is what makes it so difficult for both the patient and the health professional to recognize. Thus, a more detailed observation called the physical examination is needed.

A physical examination involves a closer inspection of the body. It focuses on specific body regions and the patient's responses to certain tests. A major sign of gonorrhea that is found during a physical examination is irritation of the genitourinary tract. This is indicated by redness of the cervix and vagina in females. Irritation of the male's urethra is very difficult to see in a normal examination, since the opening of the urethra is too small for a health-care provider to look inside. Pus from the urethra in both females and males is another indicator of gonorrhea. Any irritation like this is scrutinized as a possible STD. The CDC and other health agencies recommend that medical professionals further evaluate any condition with this sign. The following statement was produced for physicians by the CDC:

All patients who have urethritis should be evaluated for the presence of gonococcal and chlamydial infection. Testing for chlamydia is strongly recommended because of the increased utility and availability of highly sensitive and specific testing methods, and because a specific diagnosis may enhance partner notification and improve compliance with treatment, especially in the exposed partner.

Patients have to be aware that health-care providers are obligated to suspect an STD, even if this might be embarrassing to the patient.

Another important part of the patient assessment is for the health-care provider to review the patient's past medical records. These records provide a history of accidents and diseases that have been treated by health-care professionals. Medical records are confidential and are only available to approved medical professionals. Patients are allowed to see their own records, but no one else may do so. Even family members have to get permission and promise to respect the privacy of the patient before being permitted to view medical records.

The governments of many nations require that the records of certain diseases be reported confidentially or openly. Confidential reporting is used for statistical purposes to track disease trends. Gonorrhea requires confidential reporting to public health agencies and the CDC. Open reporting is needed for monitoring who may be capable of spreading dangerous communicable diseases. People diagnosed with gonorrhea may have to be identified by name to help track other people they may have infected. A person's past medical records are particularly important in identifying STDs. Many people who get STDs have a past history of being treated for the same or another STD. This is particularly true for cases of gonorrhea. The physician can use this information to counsel and educate the patient to avoid exposure to STDs in the future.

In most cases where disease is found, the physical examination is followed by a laboratory examination to confirm whether or not the patient has gonorrhea.

HOW LABORATORIES TEST FOR DISEASE

Confirming the cause of a communicable disease requires isolating and culturing the organism for positive identification. Each microbe that lives on or in the body requires a particular method of identification. Microbial isolation is a very important technique. The person testing the microbe must make sure to test a pure culture. A pure culture is a living collection of one type of organism that has not been contaminated by any other substance. Any contaminants in a culture will throw off the results of the laboratory tests used to identify gonorrhea. The testing for microbes as the cause of communicable diseases such as gonorrhea is still being perfected. It dates back to 1876 when microbiologist Robert Koch developed guidelines for confirming the cause of a communicable disease. Before his time, it was only speculated that microbes caused certain diseases. The invention of the electron microscope confirmed that microbes existed. However, it was the work of Robert Koch that allowed doctors to link a particular microbe to a certain disease. He developed a series of steps to follow to test whether a particular microbe was, in fact, causing disease in a patient. These steps became known as Koch's Postulates (see Box on page 58) and they are still used by laboratory technicians today.

LABORATORY TESTS FOR GONORRHEA

Many experimental programs have tried to find innovative ways to increase STD screening, including coupon redemption programs for free screening, home testing kits, community health fair screening, school-based programs, and routine screening in prisons and criminal detention centers.

Several tests are commercially available for the diagnosis of gonorrhea, each of which has both advantages and disadvantages:

- Culture media

- Morphology tests

- Oxidase, acid, and sucrose tests

- Enzyme substrate tests

KOCH'S POSTULATES

German bacteriologist Robert Koch came up with four steps that must be taken in determining the cause of disease. These have come to be known as "Koch's Postulates." They dictate:

1. **The pathogen must be found in all cases of the disease.** Scientists must carefully obtain samples from all suspected patients and find the same disease-causing organism present in each, if that organism is expected to be the reason for the illness.

2. **It must be isolated from the host and grown in pure culture.** The scientist must then take the pathogen and grow some of it in a laboratory, in order to have a fresh sample before going on to the next step.

3. **It must reproduce the original disease when introduced into a susceptible host.** The scientist must use the sample grown in the lab and place it (through injection, most often) into the body of a person or animal who is not immune to the disease in question. Only if the subject becomes ill with the disease can the pathogen be the cause.

4. **It must be found in the experimental host that has been infected.** That is, the scientist must then take blood or other samples from the person or animal into whom the pathogen was introduced and confirm that the original pathogen is, indeed, present, and that it is not some other organism that is causing the disease.

- Superoxol tests

- Molecular reaction tests

- Direct fluorescent antibody (DFA) tests.

Culture Media

The diagnosis of gonorrhea has traditionally been made using **culture media** (chemical mixtures designed to help bacteria or other pathogens grow in the laboratory). The culture test involves placing a sample of the patient's purulent discharge onto a culture plate and keeping it warm and safe for up to two days to allow the bacteria to multiply (Figure 4.3). *Neisseria gonorrhoeae* grows under very specific conditions using a particular medium. The medium used for *Neisseria gonorrhoeae* is made from a mixture called chocolate agar. This name comes from the fact that the medium is the same color as chocolate, due to the hemoglobin it contains. (Hemoglobin is a protein found in red blood cells. It helps the red blood cells carry oxygen throughout the blood and gives them their red color. When mixed in the medium, hemoglobin takes on a brownish color resembling chocolate.) The laboratory technicians who handle *Neisseria gonorrhoeae* must work quickly because this bacterium prefers moist environments that are low in oxygen. Too much exposure to the air can kill them.

The disadvantages of this method include this need for rapid work, along with careful transportation and storage, as well as the fact that the cultured sample takes two days to grow the bacteria, which causes a slight delay in treatment.

Morphology Test

In the laboratory, the specimen goes through a series of microbiological examinations. First, a morphology test is done to determine the shape and staining properties of the microorganism. (*Morphology* refers to the shape and growth

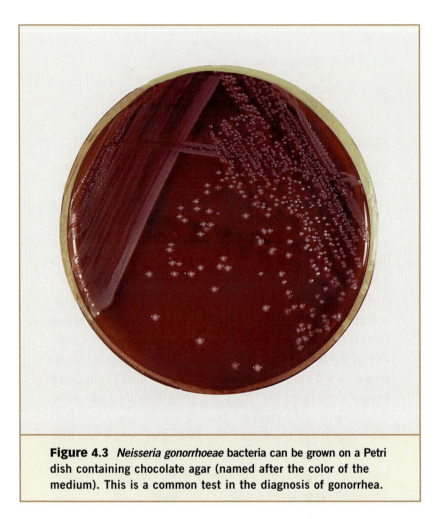

Figure 4.3 *Neisseria gonorrhoeae* bacteria can be grown on a Petri dish containing chocolate agar (named after the color of the medium). This is a common test in the diagnosis of gonorrhea.

patterns of the organism.) The overall appearance of the bacteria that grow on the culture medium is observed. *Neisseria gonorrhoeae* grows in clumps that take on a golden brown to dark pink color after growing in culture for 48 hours. Finer detail morphological testing for bacteria involves the use of Gram staining and examination under a microscope. *Neisseria gonorrhoeae* is a gram-negative bacterium and resembles spheres growing doubled up (Figure 4.4). This morphology is called "gram-negative diplococci." Most bacteria in the Neisseriaceae

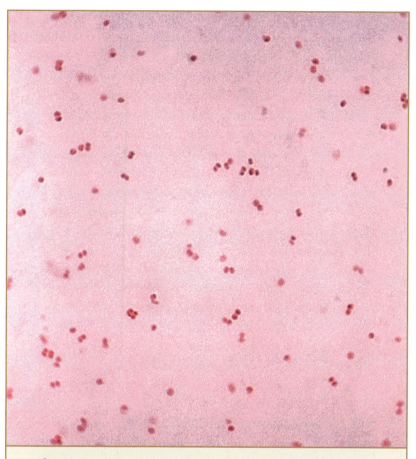

Figure 4.4 *Neisseria gonorrhoeae* bacteria have a distinct shape, and this can help with diagnosis. The bacteria are spherical, and usually grow together in pairs. This morphology (shape) is called diplococcal—*diplo* meaning "two," and *coccal* meaning "round" or "spherical."

family have this characteristic. Because of this, other tests must be done to confirm whether the bacteria in the sample are *Neisseria gonorrhoeae* or some other *Neisseria* bacterium. The next round of tests involves growing the bacteria under various conditions to analyze the characteristics of the bacteria's **metabolism**.

Oxidase, Acid, and Sucrose Tests

The oxidase test checks for the secretion of an enzyme called oxidase, a protective enzyme for *Neisseria gonorrhoeae*. Obviously, since this enzyme protects the bacterium, *Neisseria gonorrhoeae* tests positive for oxidase. Oxidase prevents oxygen from interfering with the bacterium's metabolism. As mentioned earlier, *Neisseria gonorrhoeae* is highly sensitive to oxygen.

The acid detection test evaluates how the bacteria metabolize various carbohydrates. Some bacteria produce acid waste products when they digest certain carbohydrates. *Neisseria gonorrhoeae* produces acids when it breaks down the carbohydrate glucose. It does not do this for other carbohydrates such as fructose, lactose, maltose, and sucrose.

Some bacteria will turn certain simple carbohydrates into complex chains called polymers. A procedure called the "polysaccharide from sucrose test" investigates whether the bacterium changes sucrose into a unique carbohydrate polymer. *Neisseria gonorrhoeae* converts sucrose into a starch-like chemical that turns bluish-black when mixed with iodine.

Enzyme Substrate Test

Next comes an interesting procedure called the enzyme substrate test. This technique looks for one of three enzymes produced by closely related members of the *Neisseria* family. It can tell commensal *Neisseria* apart from infections with *Neisseria gonorrhoeae*. *Neisseria gonorrhoeae* produces an enzyme called hydroxyprolyaminopeptidase. Unfortunately, certain types of the commensal *Neisseria* may produce this enzyme instead of their usual enzyme. As a result, this test alone cannot confirm the presence of *Neisseria gonorrhoeae*.

Superoxol Test

Another simple test involves adding a strong solution of hydrogen peroxide to a colony of bacteria. This is called the superoxol test. Certain bacteria, called "superoxol-positive," break down hydrogen peroxide into water and oxygen gas. The gas forms bubbles that look like foam coming out of the bacterial colony growing on the medium. *Neisseria gonorrhoeae* is superoxol-positive, so the characteristic bubbles will appear if it is present. A related test called the catalase test uses diluted hydrogen peroxide. Catalase breaks down the diluted solution into water and oxygen gas bubbles. *Neisseria gonorrhoeae* is positive for this test, too.

Testing Molecular Reactions

Other tests look at the ability of *Neisseria gonorrhoeae* to chemically react with various molecules in the environment. The nitrate reduction test looks for a metabolic pathway that converts a chemical called nitrate into a related chemical called nitrite. These are both salt-like substances commonly found in soil and water. *Neisseria gonorrhoeae* does not normally carry out this reaction. Other bacteria that can be misinterpreted as *Neisseria gonorrhoeae* are nitrate-reduction positive and do perform the reaction.

Deoxyribonuclease (DNase) is a bacterial enzyme produced to break down the **deoxyribonucleic acid** (**DNA**) that makes up an organism's genetic material. DNA is a rich source of nutrients that some bacteria are able to digest—if they secrete DNase. *Neisseria gonorrhoeae* tests negative in this procedure, which means it cannot break down DNA.

A final molecular test is performed to see if the bacteria are killed by an antibiotic called colistin sulfate. This antibiotic is similar to a chemical called colicin that is produced by intestinal bacteria. Bacteria use the chemical to reduce the growth of competing gram-negative bacteria. *Neisseria gonorrhoeae* is gram-negative but colistin sulfate does not kill it. It is referred to as "colistin resistant."

Direct Fluorescent Antibody (DFA) Tests

Direct fluorescent antibody (DFA) tests use antibodies that will appear fluorescent under an ultraviolet light when they

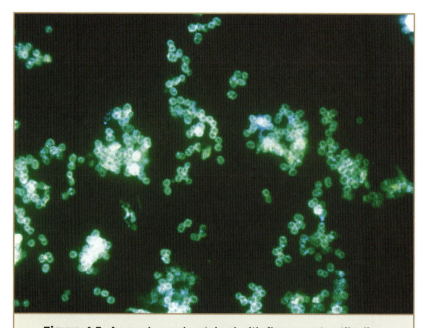

Figure 4.5 A sample can be stained with fluorescent antibodies to determine if *Neisseria gonorrhoeae* is present. This process is called a direct fluorescent antibody (DFA) test. When exposed to a fluorescent light, *Neisseria* bacteria treated in this way will glow green, as can be seen in this micrograph.

are attached to a gonorrhea bacterium (Figure 4.5). When a laboratory technician looks at the specimen through a microscope with a fluorescent light source, fluorescence indicates a positive test, meaning that *Neisseria gonorrhoeae* is present. This test is very time-consuming and relies on the expertise of the laboratory technician, so it may not be the most practical way to determine whether or not someone has gonorrhea.

REPORTING THE RESULTS

Once all the appropriate tests have been done, the medical laboratory provides a report about the results of the tests. The lab is required to compare the results of the patient's sample to a known sample of *Neisseria gonorrhoeae* and a bacterium unrelated to *Neisseria*. The *Neisseria gonorrhoeae* is called a positive control and the other bacterium is called a negative control. The patient is determined to have gonorrhea only if the patient's sample matches a correctly done positive control.

A patient who tests positive for gonorrhea is called into the health-care provider's office for special STD counseling. He or she is instructed to avoid sexual activity and is encouraged to notify all of his or her sexual partners from the past two months of his or her condition. The person is then given a single dose of antibiotic to eliminate the infection.

All positive reports of gonorrhea infection are submitted to state and federal public health agencies within a certain period of time, usually about two days after the diagnosis is made. The reports are confidential and are for data collection used in gonorrhea epidemiology studies.

THE FUTURE OF GONORRHEA DIAGNOSIS

Newer ways of testing for *Neisseria gonorrhoeae* are now being developed. The traditional tests are very slow and there is much room for error. Microbiologists are looking at instruments that identify *Neisseria gonorrhoeae* by measuring unique carbohydrates and proteins on the surface of the bacterium. The latest of these types of tests is the gonococcal antigen test. It looks for unique surface characteristics of *Neisseria gonorrhoeae*. (As you will recall from Chapter 3, antigens are proteins that provoke an immune response.) This test is approved for gonorrhea diagnosis because it has an accuracy of 88% in females and 98% in males, compared to traditional testing. Other tests are using DNA analysis to make a positive identification.

The most common DNA-based test is called the nucleic acid amplification test, or NAAT. Nucleic acid amplification tests, as the name implies, amplify the genetic building blocks (either DNA or **ribonucleic acid**, called **RNA**) rather than the organism itself. The original gonorrhea DNA or RNA can multiply as many as one billion times in just one to two hours.

This allows the test to be performed with a small number of infectious agents and on organisms that are no longer alive. As a result, the test may be used when the laboratory cannot prepare the specimen immediately for any reason.

Nucleic acid amplification tests are expensive because of the special laboratory equipment needed to perform them. In addition, nucleic acid tests take more time to properly process the specimen, but they can achieve sensitive results with fewer organisms. One of the biggest advantages of nucleic acid amplification tests is that urine specimens can be used instead of direct urethral or cervical specimens. Most patients prefer to urinate in a cup, rather than having a swab inserted into the cervix or a cotton-tipped applicator inserted into the urethra of the penis. The test results are available faster and the process is largely computerized, reducing the chance of human error causing inaccuracies.

However, DNA testing has not yet been fully approved for reporting confirmed cases of gonorrhea. Unfortunately, in 2004, five women in Hawaii tested with the NAAT method showed positive results for gonorrhea even though they did not actually have the disease. This situation is called a "false-positive" test. To prevent such errors, laboratory workers must be extremely careful when performing the NAAT.

5

Treatments and Complications of Gonorrhea

Thirty-year-old Silas goes to the doctor at the nearest medical office, complaining of burning during urination and a yellow discharge from his penis. The doctor quickly recognizes that Silas is suffering from gonorrhea. She tells Silas that the only treatment she can provide will only cure the infection in about 18% of cases, but it is all she has to offer. The doctor gives her patient the medicine, regretting the fact that she does not have other treatments available for gonorrhea because she and Silas live in a remote and poverty-stricken region of the developing African nation of Rwanda. Despite the easy cures we have for gonorrhea in the United States, Canada, and other developed countries, treatment for this widespread STD lags far behind modern medical advances in the poorer areas of the world.

Effective treatment recommendations for gonorrhea and other sexually transmitted diseases are updated by the U.S. Centers for Disease Control and Prevention (CDC) on a regular basis. You can view the current treatment guidelines online at the at the CDC Website (www.CDC.gov). To be considered a recommended treatment, the medication or technique must have a cure rate of greater than 95%. An individual case of gonorrhea is usually eliminated within 12 to 24 hours of taking a one-dose antibiotic.

THE USE OF ANTIBIOTICS

Penicillin, the first discovered antibiotic, was the first effective treatment available for gonorrhea (Figure 5.1). Dr. Alexander Fleming first discovered penicillin by accident in England in 1928. When he left his laboratory to go on vacation, Fleming forgot to put away one of his culture media plates that was growing a colony of bacteria. When he returned from his holiday, he found the plate and noticed that a mold called *Penicillium* had begun to grow on the culture medium, and that the bacteria around it had died. Fleming isolated the bacteria-killing chemical from the mold and found it to be effective in killing many different kinds of bacteria and preventing bacterial growth. Despite this revolutionary discovery, the process Fleming used to grow the bacteria-killing chemical—which he named "penicillin" after the mold from which it came—produced enough for laboratory experiments but not enough to treat even a single patient with a bacterial illness. Because of this difficulty, penicillin was largely ignored until the United States entered World War II in 1941.

WHAT IS THE CDC?

The Centers for Disease Control and Prevention (CDC) is a branch of the Department of Health and Human Services, part of the U.S. federal government. The main headquarters of the CDC is located in Atlanta, Georgia. The major responsibilities of the CDC are to protect the health and safety of people at home and abroad, to provide a source of information so that the general public and health-care providers can make decisions based on strong scientific evidence, and to promote health through strong partnerships within communities and with other countries. The CDC Website—http://www.cdc.gov—is an excellent resource for health information and current trends in the incidence of all types of diseases, from anthrax to the flu.

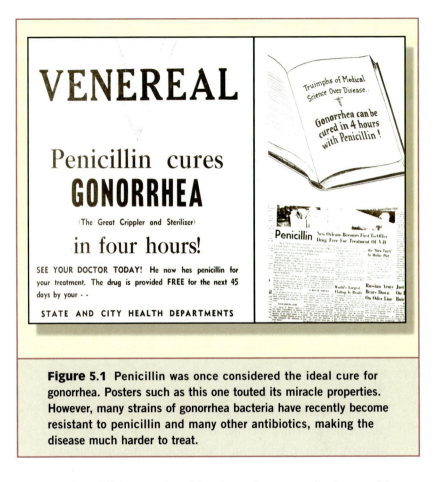

Figure 5.1 Penicillin was once considered the ideal cure for gonorrhea. Posters such as this one touted its miracle properties. However, many strains of gonorrhea bacteria have recently become resistant to penicillin and many other antibiotics, making the disease much harder to treat.

In addition to the risk of gunshot wounds that could become infected, soldiers were also exposed to poor sanitary conditions while on the warfront. To help save the lives of soldiers at the hand of infections (rather than enemy troops), the U.S. government recognized the potential value of penicillin and poured enormous financial and scientific resources into researching ways to mass-produce penicillin to treat bacterial disease. By the end of World War II, production of penicillin had increased 2,500-fold. As you will recall from Chapter 2, penicillin was so effective against gonorrhea that many people mistakenly came to believe that the disease had been eliminated for good. But this was not true. Besides the more relaxed sexual practices of the 1960s and 1970s, gonorrhea continued to be a health threat for another very important reason—its growing ability to resist being killed by certain antibiotics.

DEVELOPMENT OF ANTIBIOTIC RESISTANCE

Gonorrhea easily develops resistance to antibiotics. This resistance has been a serious deterrent to the effectiveness of disease control programs. The first case of antibiotic resistance in gonorrhea developed in the 1940s very shortly after penicillin was first introduced. Although it was once the mainstay of gonorrhea treatment, penicillin has now been removed from the CDC's list of recommended treatments for gonorrhea. Resistance patterns are different in other areas of the world, however, and penicillin is still considered a very effective treatment for gonorrhea in some places, like England, for example. Overall, 18% of tested gonorrhea specimens are resistant to penicillin, tetracycline (another antibiotic), or both. This ability to develop resistance is an essential survival feature of the *Neisseria gonorrhoeae* bacterium.

Antibiotic resistance in gonorrhea develops in two ways. Any single gonorrhea bacterium may employ one or both techniques to protect itself from destruction. In the first method, the gonorrhea bacterium prevents the antibiotic from getting to its target site, either by actively removing the antibiotic from the cell by means of pumps, or by producing enzymes that destroy the antibiotic before it gets to its target. These enzymes are only effective against the antibiotics penicillin and tetracycline. The second method of developing antibiotic resistance is to alter the target site on the gonorrhea so that antibiotics are not effective. This occurs through a change made during the bacterium's reproduction process in the proteins of the cell wall of the bacterium, so that the antibiotic is unable to penetrate it. This change in the bacterium's cell wall that stops one antibiotic may prevent another antibiotic from killing it as well.

The spread of antibiotic resistance occurs because gonorrhea changes its genetic makeup to try to survive when it comes in contact with an antibiotic. When the bacteria becomes resistant, the infection is not cured and can continue to be spread to other people through sexual contact. These people, too, will be infected with resistant strains of gonorrhea, making the disease more and more difficult to treat.

WHICH ANTIBIOTIC TO USE

The portal of entry and the severity of the disease determine the type of antibiotic therapy a doctor will choose to treat a case of gonorrhea. The CDC refers to a simple gonorrhea infection that was acquired recently as an "uncomplicated gonococcal infection." Such cases are treated with one of several specific antibiotics. Different dosages of the antibiotics are used for pregnant women, to avoid harming the fetus. A single 400-mg oral dose of cefixime is enough to provide a 97–99% cure rate for "uncomplicated" gonorrhea. Other oral single-dose antibiotic treatments include ciprofloxacin, levofloxicin, norfloxicin, and ofloxicin. These four antibiotics are chemically classified as "**quinolones**." Unfortunately, certain types of *Neisseria gonorrhoeae* are resistant to quinolones, making the drugs ineffective.

Another useful treatment is a single shot of ceftriaxone, cefotaximine, or spectinomycin injected into the muscle, called an "intramuscular injection," abbreviated "IM." These are very effective but can be quite painful.

Pharyngeal gonorrhea is controlled with ceftriaxone, ciprofloxacin, or bactrim DS. Disseminated gonorrhea (recall Marie's case from Chapter 4) requires long-term therapy. Intravenous (IV) antibiotics must be given for 7 to 10 days. An intravenous injection is administered through a needle directly into a vein. Other treatments use the standard oral or intramuscular injection, given repeatedly until all evidence of the disease is gone. Most of these treatments require that the patient remain in the hospital until he or she tests negative for gonorrhea. Public health officials discourage outpatient therapy for disseminated gonorrhea. (*Outpatient* means that the infected person visits the hospital only for the treatment and then returns home.) Data show that many people do not return for subsequent treatment if permitted to leave the hospital. This encourages the development of antibiotic resistant bacteria.

All treatments for gonorrhea require a follow-up medical examination. The time of the visit to the doctor varies, depending on the type of treatment used and how severe the case of gonorrhea was. Usually, patients are asked to return for a follow-up exam one to two months after treatment. The follow-up consists of the same testing used for the initial diagnosis. Disseminated gonorrhea may require a more intensive medical examination to evaluate how well damaged body parts have healed. After this follow-up, the patient is encouraged to make regular visits to a medical professional to ensure a full return to health.

COMPLICATIONS

If left untreated, gonorrhea can cause a multitude of problems, some of which can progress to serious and even life-threatening illnesses.

Epididymitis

Epididymitis, or inflammation of the epididymis, is the most common local complication of gonorrhea in males. The **epididymis** is a duct that transports sperm from the testicle to the vas deferens, the tube that connects the testes with the urethra. Epididymitis causes a painful swelling of the scrotum, testicular pain, or tenderness. The pain may be mild, or may be severe enough to make walking difficult. Epididymitis may be the first sign of a gonorrhea infection, or it may be preceded by burning with urination. The onset of pain may be sudden or gradual.

Bartholin's Gland Abscess

Females with gonorrhea may develop an abscess of the Bartholin's gland, a tiny organ located at the opening of the vagina that is invisible to the naked eye. This gland functions as a source of lubrication for the vaginal lips. When an abscess develops, the blocked duct becomes very painful and may swell to such an extent that it restricts the woman's ability to walk. To treat this condition, a doctor will usually remove the abscess with a scalpel and place a temporary drain in the duct to keep it open. Oral antibiotics are prescribed to eliminate the infection.

Pelvic Inflammatory Disease

Pelvic inflammatory disease (PID), an infection of the upper genital tract, is a life-threatening and, unfortunately, common complication of gonorrhea among women. It involves the fallopian tubes, uterus, and ovaries, and occurs in approximately 10% to 17% of females who get gonorrhea. The incidence of PID is difficult to track because doctors are not required to report it to local health departments, and most infections these days do not require the patient to be hospitalized. It is estimated that about 20% of all PID cases occur among adolescent females.

PID begins in the cervix and ascends to the lining of the uterus and to the fallopian tubes, ovaries, and abdomen. The abdominal cavity contains the lower portion of the digestive system, including the intestines, liver, pancreas, spleen, and stomach. A delicate membrane called the peritoneum lines the abdominal cavity and surrounds all of these organs. It is probable that *Neisseria gonorrhoeae* could leave the fallopian tubes and start growing on the peritoneum. This is followed by inflammation and perforation of the delicate membrane. (A perforation is a hole in the membrane that then exposes the internal organs to possible hazards, including pathogenic microbes.) After the peritoneum is perforated, all of the organs are vulnerable to destruction by *Neisseria gonorrhoeae.*

Liver infections occur in 15–20% of PID cases. PID is so painful and debilitating that it usually forces people to seek a health-care provider's care. However, medical treatments can do little more than kill the bacteria to stop them from causing further destruction—they cannot normally reverse any damage that has already been done.

The most common symptom of PID is lower abdominal pain. Other symptoms include a mucopurulent vaginal discharge, pain during sexual intercourse, dysuria (burning with urination), nausea, vomiting, and fever. PID caused by gonorrhea is believed to cause more severe symptoms than PID that results from chlamydia infection.

The diagnosis of PID is made through a clinical pelvic examination by a health-care provider. In the first part of the exam, a plastic or metal instrument called a speculum is inserted into the vagina, allowing the health-care provider to look inside the vagina and cervix. Samples are taken from the cervix with cotton-tipped applicators to check for sexually transmitted diseases. A bimanual exam follows the speculum exam and is essential for making the diagnosis of PID. Two gloved fingers are inserted into the vagina, then pressure is applied to the lower part of the abdomen. The clinician moves the cervix from side to side, which puts pressure on the fallopian tubes and will cause pain if the tubes are inflamed. The uterus is then pushed from below by the fingers in the vagina and from above by the hand on the abdomen. A report of tenderness when the uterus or cervix is moved in this manner constitutes the minimal criterion needed to make a diagnosis of PID.

Prompt and complete treatment of PID is important because the infection can result in scarring of the fallopian tubes. When scarring occurs, the egg may not be able to pass through the tube to enter the uterus during ovulation, resulting in infertility, or the inability to become pregnant. Alternatively, the egg may become fertilized but may not be

able to pass into the uterus to grow. In this situation, called **ectopic pregnancy**, the egg usually attaches to the fallopian tube, where it cannot grow normally (see Box on page 80). This type of pregnancy is life-threatening to the mother and almost always fatal to the fetus. Women with a history of PID have 3 to 10 times more of a risk of ectopic pregnancy.

Whether a woman will be left infertile by an episode of pelvic inflammatory disease (PID) depends on the severity of the damage to the fallopian tubes. This can only be determined through **laparoscopy**, which is not routinely done to diagnosis PID because the procedure itself can be risky. There is a 3% infertility rate when there is only mild tube involvement during a PID infection, a 13% rate when there is moderate damage, and a 29% rate with severe damage. The severity of the symptoms during a PID infection does not correlate with the amount of damage observed; for example, the existence of mild symptoms does not mean that there is only minimal internal damage. Infertility is an end result of a complex process of infection, inflammation, and tissue repair. Each recurrent episode of PID increases the risk of infertility, with 8% rates of infertility after one episode, 20% after two, and 40% after three or more occurrences.

Human Immunodeficiency Virus (HIV)

People with gonorrhea can more easily contract human immunodeficiency virus (HIV), the virus that causes AIDS. The process for increased transmission of HIV is unclear but is believed to be related to the inflammatory effects of gonorrhea. The inflammation brings target cells for HIV to the mucous membrane surfaces, increasing the likelihood of transmission. HIV acquisition is up to five times higher when the person infected with gonorrhea has sexual intercourse with an HIV-infected partner as compared to those who do not have gonorrhea. Transmission of HIV is also higher from a person with both HIV and gonorrhea. The viral load (number of viruses) of HIV in the semen of infected men with gonorrhea is eight times higher than in those without gonorrhea. The more virus that is present, the higher the transmission risk.

Disseminated Gonorrhea Infection (DGI)

Disseminated gonorrhea infection (DGI), like Marie's case from Chapter 4, is the spread of gonorrhea to parts of the body beyond the genitourinary tract. Fortunately, DGI is rare, occurring in just 0.2% to 1.9% of all infections of the mucous membranes. The human immune system is usually able to prevent the gonorrhea bacteria from circulating beyond the

GONOCOCCAL ISOLATE SURVEILLANCE PROJECT (GISP)

GISP is a CDC-sponsored surveillance system that was established in 1986. The project monitors antibiotic susceptibility in gonorrhea to determine the most effective treatment approaches. Five thousand male urethral gonorrhea specimens are obtained each year from 27 cities across the United States. These centers send the first 25 positive cultures from men to the project each month. Demographic and clinical data are included for each specimen. All the specimens are tested to see how susceptible they are to penicillin, tetracycline, spectinomycin, ciprofloxacin, ceftriaxone, cefixime, and azithromycin. The information obtained is used to chart antibiotic resistance patterns and help guide treatment recommendations in the United States (Figure 5.2). The information from the United States is reported to the WHO, along with data from European countries, Latin America, the Caribbean, the Western Pacific, and Southeast Asia, to monitor information on antibiotic susceptibility and information on trends in new resistance.

mucous membranes. DGI is much more common among women than men. For every man who gets the condition, four women suffer from DGI.

Certain strains of gonorrhea are more likely than others to lead to DGI. Scientists believe that these strains may be more resistant to the killing action of the normal immune system, but fortunately, are more sensitive to penicillin.

The symptoms of DGI begin with a mild feeling of illness and fever up to 102.2°F (39°C). Two-thirds of patients will have joint pain, either in one or multiple joints. The wrists, fingers, knees, and ankles are the most commonly affected

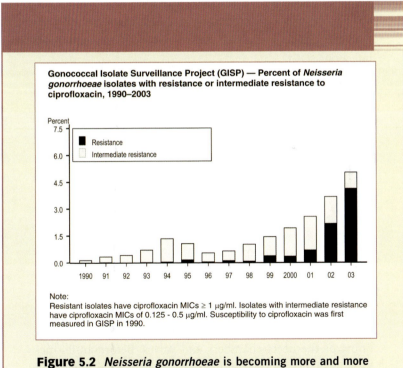

Gonococcal Isolate Surveillance Project (GISP) — Percent of *Neisseria gonorrhoeae* isolates with resistance or intermediate resistance to ciprofloxacin, 1990–2003

Note:
Resistant isolates have ciprofloxacin MICs ≥ 1 µg/ml. Isolates with intermediate resistance have ciprofloxacin MICs of 0.125 - 0.5 µg/ml. Susceptibility to ciprofloxacin was first measured in GISP in 1990.

Figure 5.2 *Neisseria gonorrhoeae* is becoming more and more resistant to antibiotics, as can be seen in this graph. This makes gonorrhea harder to treat and leaves doctors with fewer treatment options for their patients.

joints. Once they enter the closed space of a joint, the bacteria can trigger an acute (rapid-onset) inflammation in just a few hours. This may lead to fast destruction of the joint and bone loss, and the victim may ultimately lose the ability to use the joint.

Another classic symptom of DGI is a skin rash, or dermatitis, that is usually seen along with the joint pain. The dermatitis appears as tender, necrotic sores with a red base (Figure 5.3). The rash occurs below the neck and is most likely to be found on the lower parts of extremities. There may be anywhere from 5 to 40 individual sores that go away in 4 to 5 days without leaving any scarring.

The infection responds quickly to antibiotics, with complete recovery happening within a few days. Intravenous treatment with ceftriaxone is necessary to treat disseminated gonorrhea infections (DGI).

Interestingly, alternative medicine treatments for disseminated gonorrhea have been used with some success. One treatment involves a 10-day course of a combination of acupuncture, garlic, pricking blood, cupping (affecting blood flow by placing suction cups on the skin), and removing fluid from the joints. This regimen was used in a research study of 116 patients with gonococcal arthritis. Of the total number of patients, 64% were cured. To date, no other complementary or alternative medicine treatments has been found to be effective in treating gonorrhea infections.

Endocarditis

Gonorrhea rarely travels to infect the heart, but when it does, the result is **endocarditis**, an inflammation of the interior lining of the heart chambers and valves. Before antibiotics were available to treat gonorrhea, endocarditis accounted for 26% of all cases of DGI. Since the advent of antibiotics, endocarditis occurs in fewer than 2% of all cases of DGI. Men are more commonly affected than women. The symptoms of

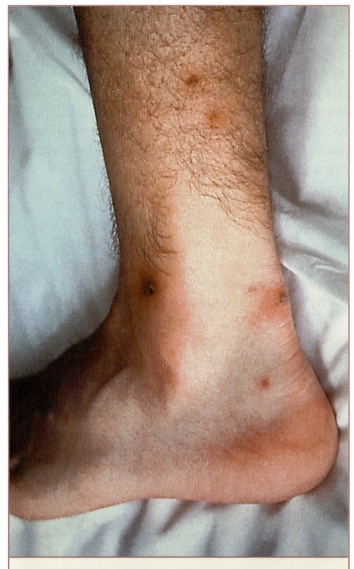

Figure 5.3 Occasionally, gonorrhea can spread to the skin, a condition called disseminated gonorrhea infection (DGI). DGI can cause a rash and/or skin lesions, as seen on the man's leg in this photograph. Although the patient must be treated with intravenous antibiotics, the condition is curable and usually does not leave any scars.

ECTOPIC PREGNANCY

Ectopic pregnancy is the leading cause of death for women during the first three months of pregnancy. Fortunately, these deaths are extremely rare because health-care providers are able to recognize the signs of an ectopic pregnancy. The symptoms include cramping and spotting early in the pregnancy, and the pain gradually increases to severe lower abdominal pain on one side of the body.

gonoccocal endocarditis include a fever with spikes in the temperature twice a day. Other symptoms include joint pain, rapid heartbeat, fatigue, and congestive heart failure. There is a 75% survival rate for this infection. More than 50% of the cases require a surgical valve replacement to save the patient's life.

Prostate Cancer

New research shows a link between a history of a gonorrhea infection and the development of prostate cancer. In a large study that was designed to find out why black males develop prostate cancer at twice the rate of white males, researchers found that 65% of men with prostate cancer had a history of gonorrhea, compared with 53% of those without prostate cancer. The men with cancer were also more likely to have had gonorrhea more than once. An exact cause-and-effect relationship cannot yet be made between gonorrhea and prostate cancer, but research is continuing to explore how the two diseases might be connected.

6

Gonorrhea in the World Today

According to the World Health Organization (WHO), 62 million new gonorrhea infections are diagnosed each year. This represents only about half of all annual gonorrhea infections, because many infections are treated without testing and others are asymptomatic and are never diagnosed or treated. Gonorrhea is the second most frequently reported communicable disease in the United States, after infection with human papillomavirus (HPV), the cause of genital warts. Although the rate of gonorrhea has decreased by 73% since 1975 (most likely due to safer sex practices that occurred with the start of the HIV/AIDS epidemic in the early 1980s), recent data shows that this trend is reversing itself, especially among adolescents and men who have sex with men.

Epidemiologists use the term *prevalence* to describe the number of people carrying a particular disease at a particular moment. Prevalence can only be calculated if the disease is diagnosed and recorded in some type of database. The Centers for Disease Control and Prevention (CDC) and the World Health Organization (WHO) keep track of disease prevalence globally and individually for each country. Other terms that are important to epidemiologists are *endemic, epidemic,* and *pandemic. Endemic* refers to a disease that is limited to a small population of people living in a particular region, but is always present to some extent. Colds are endemic in many areas because they spread within communities as people make regular daily contact with each other. A large number of cases dispersed across various geographic regions makes up an *epidemic.*

A *pandemic* is a worldwide outbreak of a disease. Gonorrhea usually appears as an endemic disease and is localized to a particular population engaged in high-risk sexual activity. However, its association with AIDS is making gonorrhea a pandemic disease.

GONORRHEA IN DEVELOPING NATIONS

Throughout the world, the most socially or economically marginalized people have the highest rates of gonorrhea and other sexually transmitted diseases. The poorest people lack access to good medical care, including diagnosis and treatment of diseases. In poor countries, whatever medical resources exist must be used first to combat immediate life-threatening health problems, such as starvation and malnutrition. In these nations (as you will recall from the story of Silas in Chapter 5), antibiotics are not readily available for many diseases, including STDs. It has been estimated that the cost of effective treatment

WHAT IS THE WORLD HEALTH ORGANIZATION (WHO)?

The WHO is a single global health organization formed in 1945. It was founded to initiate and coordinate public health campaigns around the world. The WHO was the first organization to define "health" not just as the absence of disease but as the promotion of physical, mental, and social well-being. The WHO has attempted to decrease the differences between those people in the world with access to health-care systems and healthy lifestyles and those without. The WHO's job is to monitor disease incidence and prevalence and to keep track of the spread of infections in nations across the world. The WHO was responsible for the elimination of smallpox through an intensive worldwide vaccination program. The last natural case of smallpox occurred in 1977 in Somalia.

for gonorrhea in Africa would be equal to half the current health budget of the entire continent.

GONORRHEA IN DEVELOPED NATIONS

The United States has the highest rate of gonorrhea of any industrialized country in the world. The rate is 50 times greater than that of Sweden and 8 times greater than Canada's, especially among teenagers. Interestingly, teen sexual activity rates are about the same in all industrialized countries, but the sexually transmitted disease and unplanned pregnancy rates are much higher in the United States. This discrepancy is explained by several behavioral and social factors. Teenagers in the United States are more likely than those in other developed countries to have two or more sexual partners. U.S. teenagers are also less likely to use a condom.

In the United States, the highest incidence of gonorrhea is among adolescent females between the ages of 15 and 19, followed by females 20–24 years old and then males 20–24 years old (Figure 6.1). At all ages, females are more likely to acquire gonorrhea than males, because females have more mucous membranes in the genital area for the bacteria to infect. Gonorrhea rates are highest in the southern parts of the United States (Figure 6.2). Racial disparities exist for most medical problems, and gonorrhea is no exception. The incidence of gonorrhea among African Americans is 30 times higher than the rate among whites (Figure 6.3). There are many factors that account for this disproportionate rate. The first of these is a reporting bias; poverty and lack of medical insurance results in a greater proportion of African Americans seeking care in public clinics, which report gonorrhea at higher rates than private medical offices do.

RISK FACTORS

The number of lifetime sexual partners is a risk factor for becoming infected with gonorrhea and other STDs. Those

ALCOHOL, DRUGS, AND STDS

Experimentation, rebellion, and youth go together in many societies. The rebellion of youth sometimes drives teens to experiment with alcohol, drugs, and sex. This interrelationship is highly evident when investigating the epidemiology of sexually transmitted diseases. In many regions of the world, alcohol and drug abuse are major causative factors in homicides, motor vehicle accidents, and suicides. Recent studies on data collected over many years show that substance abuse also results in a higher incidence of acquiring STDs. The problem of alcohol abuse and STDs has become so important that the National Institute on Alcohol Abuse and Alcoholism (NIAAA) released a public alert about the problem in 2000. NIAAA is a part of the National Institutes of Health (NIH), headquartered in Bethesda, Maryland. The NIAAA data suggest that people who abuse alcohol are more likely to engage in high-risk sexual behaviors, including unprotected sex and sexual contact with partners who are at risk of having STDs. High-risk partners include injection-drug users, people who have multiple sexual partners, and prostitutes. Data from other studies conducted at NIH find the same correlation between drug abuse and STDs. Although AIDS was the primary focus of the study, the data hold true for gonorrhea and other common STDs as well. With this information, healthcare providers are becoming vigilant about educating people about this risk. Teens and young adults are the most likely group to engage in high-risk sexual activity while under the influence of alcohol or drugs. It is not surprising to learn that the CDC has reported that higher alcohol taxes and higher minimum legal drinking ages implemented between 1981 and 1995 have been associated with a decline STD incidence among adolescents.

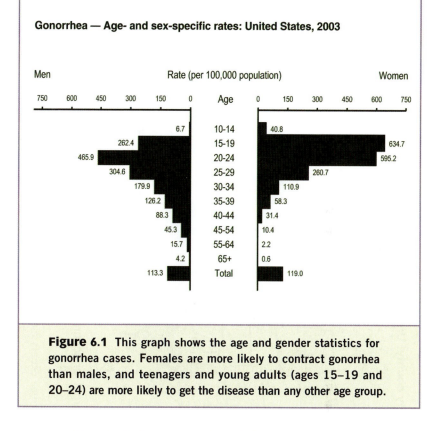

Gonorrhea — Age- and sex-specific rates: United States, 2003

Figure 6.1 This graph shows the age and gender statistics for gonorrhea cases. Females are more likely to contract gonorrhea than males, and teenagers and young adults (ages 15–19 and 20–24) are more likely to get the disease than any other age group.

people with the highest number of lifetime partners have the highest incidence of STDs. Additionally, the more partners a person has within a short period of time, the higher the risk for STDs. This is because such people are likely having sexual intercourse with people they may not know very well. These sexual partners are also more likely to have engaged in sexual intercourse with multiple partners, which further compounds the risk.

Adolescents at Risk

Three million adolescents get an STD each year. To truly appreciate the incidence of STDs among adolescents, you need to

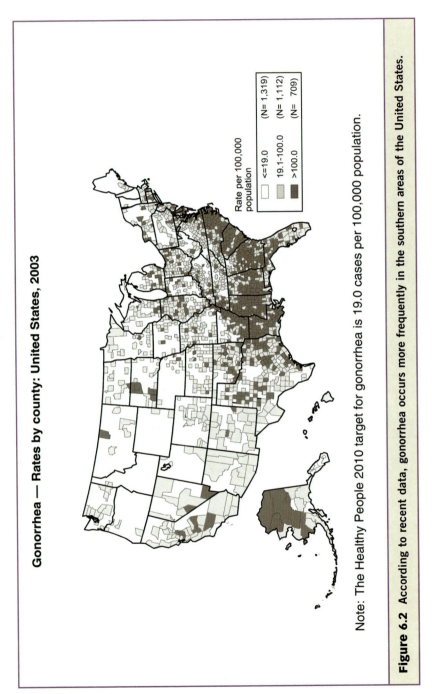

Gonorrhea — Rates by county: United States, 2003

Rate per 100,000 population

<=19.0	(N= 1,319)
19.1-100.0	(N= 1,112)
>100.0	(N= 709)

Note: The Healthy People 2010 target for gonorrhea is 19.0 cases per 100,000 population.

Figure 6.2 According to recent data, gonorrhea occurs more frequently in the southern areas of the United States.

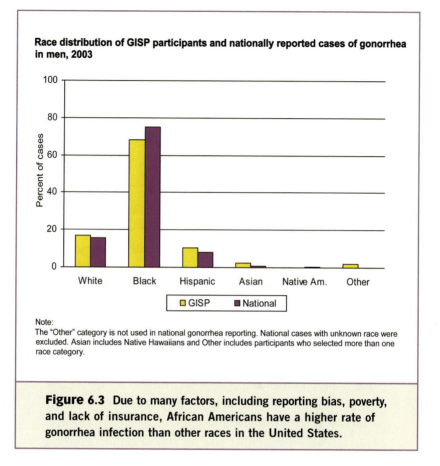

Race distribution of GISP participants and nationally reported cases of gonorrhea in men, 2003

Note:
The "Other" category is not used in national gonorrhea reporting. National cases with unknown race were excluded. Asian includes Native Hawaiians and Other includes participants who selected more than one race category.

Figure 6.3 Due to many factors, including reporting bias, poverty, and lack of insurance, African Americans have a higher rate of gonorrhea infection than other races in the United States.

remember that the STD rate is usually recorded in rates per 1,000 people. Of these 1,000 adolescents, only about half may be sexually active. This is a much higher rate than those recorded among 1,000 adults, of whom most are sexually active. There are many factors that place adolescents at increased risk to acquire an STD and can be divided into biological, behavioral, and social risk factors.

Biological Risk Factors

Biological risk factors can be attributed to the cellular changes that occur in the cervix as a young woman matures. Until young adulthood, the surface of the cervix is made up of what are called columnar epithelial cells; as the young woman grows, these cells are replaced by squamous cells. Columnar cells are much more susceptible to STD infection. Another biological risk factor is the immature local immunity and low number of antibodies to STDs among most young people. Because of these factors, a teen's contact with gonorrhea is more likely to result in an infection.

Behavioral Risk Factors

Behavioral risk factors have to do with the things young people may do that make them more susceptible to gonorrhea. Adolescents have higher rates of infections with no symptoms; therefore, they are less likely than adults to seek treatment. In addition, they are frequently unaware that many infections may be asymptomatic and therefore falsely assume that it is safe to have sexual intercourse without a condom if the partner does not show any symptoms of disease. Other behavioral risk factors for the acquisition of STDs include multiple sexual partners and inconsistent condom use. Adolescents report that they do not use condoms because they believe their sexual partners will react negatively to the request for the use of a condom. They would rather take the risk of getting a disease than risk rejection from a partner. Sexual intercourse without a condom is mistakenly seen as an indication of love and loyalty.

Social Risk Factors

Social risk factors are related to barriers to access to health care for adolescents. Without prompt diagnosis and treatment of infections, the infected partner pool gets larger. Adolescents may not seek care because of fear that their parents or guardians will be notified of the results of the testing. Since 1975, in all 50 states and the District of Columbia, adolescents have been able to obtain confidential testing and treatment for sexually transmitted diseases. Yet only about one-third of

WHERE DO YOU STAND ON CONFI-DENTIAL CARE FOR ADOLESCENTS?

The principle of confidentiality limits the disclosure of medical information and protects the privacy of patients. The extent of the rights of adolescents to confidential care varies from state to state. In all states, adolescents are able to receive assessment and treatment for STDs confidentially, and in many states, there are specific laws that allow adolescents to receive birth control without their parents' knowledge and consent. Since the 1970s, laws have prohibited federally funded clinics from requiring parental consent before providing contraceptive services to minors. These laws are often controversial. People have very different opinions on whether it is wise to give minors the right to consent and confidentiality when it comes to sexual matters.

People who oppose giving adolescents the right to seek and receive contraceptive services and other reproductive health care believe that parental involvement encourages abstinence. The thinking goes that, if adolescents have to ask a parent for permission to get birth control or have an STD screening, they are less likely to have sex. Opponents of confidential care believe that required parental consent will increase communication between parents and their teenagers about contraception that could convince young people to abstain from sexual activity or increase their likelihood of safe-sex practices. Opponents of confidential care also believe it is the right of parents to make all health-care decisions for their underage children.

Advocates of confidential care believe it is essential for encouraging openness between the health-care specialist and the adolescent patient. They argue that, without this trust, the adolescent will not provide complete and accurate information and the health-care provider will not be aware of the patient's potential risks for STDs and unplanned pregnancy. The proponents of confidential care believe confidentiality improves access to health care for adolescents.

adolescents are aware of this legal right. Access to care is also limited because adolescents are often uninsured or under-insured, and are unable to pay for the services they need for STD diagnosis and treatment.

Who Is at Risk?

Specific groups of adolescents are at increased risk; those in the juvenile justice system have the highest rate, probably because of a clustering of risk factors. Any adolescent with a history of ever having had a STD is more likely to contract another STD. Homeless and runaway youths are at increased risk of all STDs because of a lack of medical care for themselves and their partner pool. Trading sex for money and shelter also puts these young people at risk. Gay and lesbian youths also have higher rates of sexually transmitted diseases. These adolescents tend to have an earlier age of sexual initiation and engage in higher-risk sexual activity with multiple partners and without condoms.

Because gonorrhea can lead to some devastating conse-quences if not properly treated, it is essential for all people—and teens in particular—to understand the disease and help stop its spread.

7

The Future of Gonorrhea

"If I tried to paint a symbolic picture of syphilis control in our contemporary American scene, I would show a few green islands of intelligent activity, a good many sand bars of effort, and the whole surrounded by the vast gray waters of apathy, futility, and ignorance." These words were spoken by U.S. Surgeon General Thomas Parran about syphilis in the 1930s. Unfortunately, his statement remains just as true for gonorrhea in the 21st century as it was for syphilis in the early 20th century.

It is estimated that the United States spends $1 billion annually on the treatment of gonorrhea infections and its complications. Because of the higher rates of gonorrhea among teens, prevention strategies are focused on the adolescent population at both the individual and societal levels. The three critical elements of STD prevention include:

1. Decreasing the transmissibility of the disease

2. Decreasing the length of time an individual is infected

3. Decreasing the number of sexual contacts.

PREVENTING GONORRHEA

Public health officials all agree that preventing gonorrhea is much better than treating the disease. Obviously, the safest and simplest prevention is to avoid all types of sexual contact. However, this is not always desirable or practical. So, health-care providers suggest that sexual contact be kept to one individual who is at a low risk for contracting STDs. Sexually active people should have regular checkups that include STD testing. This should include the testing of every partner in a sexual relationship.

Avoiding alcohol and illicit drugs before sexual activity is also important. Alcohol and drugs can lead to impaired judgment that puts a person at risk for STDs. Avoiding sexual activities with drug abusers and prostitutes also reduces the chance of contracting gonorrhea and other STDs.

Safer Sex

Safer sex (using a condom) is the next recommended method for reducing the incidence of gonorrhea and other STDs. Condoms (Figure 7.1a), if used consistently and correctly, are an effective way to ward off gonorrhea. The condom must fit properly to avoid leakage and prevent any direct contact with the partner's body. Condoms should be used for any type of sexual activity—whether vaginal, oral, or anal—in order to be fully effective. Female condoms (Figure 7.1b) are also available. They are made of rubber-like material shaped like a sack that fits snugly in the vagina. Again, these must be used properly to reduce the risk of contracting STDs. (Male and female condoms cannot be used at the same time.) Diaphragms, herbal extracts, lubricants, sponges, vaginal spermicides, and birth control pills designed to prevent pregnancy are useless for protecting against STDs. Some of these products actually irritate the vaginal lining, making it more vulnerable than it normally would be to gonorrhea and other STDs. Certain substances should never be used with condoms as a way to prevent STDs. The chemicals used to make these products can break down the condom. The condom can actually be weakened enough to allow pathogens to pass through the latex and cause infection.

Abstinence

Postponing sexual activity, or **abstinence,** helps control the spread of gonorrhea by decreasing the number of sexual partners a person has during his or her lifetime. Over the last few decades, the age of the average first experience with sexual

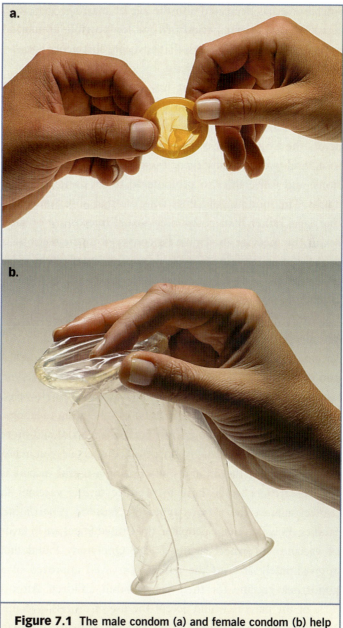

Figure 7.1 The male condom (a) and female condom (b) help protect against pregnancy and many sexually transmitted diseases, including gonorrhea.

intercourse has decreased and the age of marriage increased, resulting in a longer period of time for possible premarital sexual intercourse. Programs that advocate abstinence encourage teens to delay sexual activity.

The federal government has appropriated millions of dollars through Maternal and Child Health Block Grants to develop abstinence-only education programs in communities across the United States. These grants provide funding at the local level to community agencies, schools, religious organizations, and universities to promote abstinence among young adults. The funding guidelines stipulate that abstinence until marriage, rather than postponing sexual intercourse or safer sex, is the message that must be conveyed to the teens. It is too early to determine if these programs are effective, since the few published evaluations of these programs have shown conflicting results.

Vaccination

Vaccination is not yet a preventative option for gonorrhea and other STDs. The only vaccine that has shown success in laboratory tests has not yet been tested in humans. However, nasal applications of an experimental vaccine given to laboratory mice protected them against gonorrhea. More and more studies are being conducted to produce effective gonorrhea vaccines. Part of the difficulty in creating a useful vaccine is that researchers would have to produce several vaccines to protect against the various types of *Neisseria gonorrhoeae*. Studies show that many people in the United States are in favor of vaccines to protect against STDs. One study found that approximately 76% of the parents surveyed approved of a gonorrhea vaccine for their young adult children. Almost 90% of the parents would accept the use of an HIV vaccine, and the idea of a genital herpes vaccine was also popular. The major problem with vaccines is that they are not always 100% effective and may require follow-up vaccinations called boosters every few years. Many people do not request vaccinations because they are financially unable to afford the treatment. Plus, many people who are at risk for contracting various diseases may be uneducated about the benefits of vaccinations.

EDUCATION STRATEGIES

Many public health strategies to prevent the spread of STDs consist of education about the disease, especially education directed toward adolescents. Single-focused educational strategies (such as programs that emphasize abstinence only and do not teach about safer sex techniques) have been shown in some studies to be ineffective, because without an appreciation of risk, behavior will not change, despite knowledge of possible harm. Teens often think they will never be affected by negative

VACCINE ACCEPTANCE: WHERE DO YOU STAND?

Do you believe that fear of STDs encourages abstinence and monogamy? Some people believe that vaccines for STDs should not be available because the acquisition of an STD is an effective punishment for sexual behavior that is seen as morally wrong. In addition, some believe that if the risk of acquiring an STD is gone, people will engage in more promiscuous sexual behavior.

If there were a vaccine for gonorrhea, at what age do you think it should be given to people? To be an effective prevention strategy, the vaccine would have to be administered before sexual activity begins. Will doctors and parents be comfortable vaccinating school-age children against sexually transmitted diseases? The idea of vaccination against gonorrhea and other STDs is an acknowledgment that there is a risk of contracting an STD. Will parents be comfortable accepting that their children are at risk and consent to vaccination?

events such as accidents or disease. Strategies already in place to prevent pregnancy can be coordinated with prevention of STDs, since both are consequences of unprotected sexual intercourse. In countries with lower teenage pregnancy and STD rates, comprehensive sexuality education, not abstinence promotion, is emphasized. The goal of comprehensive education is to provide information and demonstrate responsible decision-making rather than focusing solely on the prevention of sexual intercourse. Positive attitudes about sexuality with clear expectations about appropriate and safe behavior have resulted in more responsible teenage sexual activity, which extends through adulthood in these countries.

SKILL BUILDING

Strategies that add skill building to the educational component of sexuality education have been shown to be effective. These skills include improving communication skills to help postpone sexual involvement or, if the young person is already sexually active, to communicate the need to use a condom to his or her sexual partners. Programs that improve life options for adolescents have demonstrated success in pregnancy and disease prevention. The sense of future is improved for adolescents in poor areas by increasing their feelings of connectedness to school, offering opportunities for future careers through educational achievement, and providing structured time for teen recreation and more interaction with responsible adults.

Adolescents in the United States often receive conflicting messages about sexual behavior. The reality of life in our modern culture is that teens are constantly exposed to sexual imagery through a large variety of media outlets, including television, movies, music videos, computer games, and the Internet. Teens are told to abstain from sexual intercourse at the same time that they are bombarded with images of provocative sexual situations. The use of condoms and other forms of contraception is rarely shown in the media, and the negative

EATING RIGHT TO AVOID STDS

People today often take it for granted that most diseases are easily cured with a pill or an injection. Even better is the feeling that taking a vaccine every few years can simply prevent most diseases in the first place. However, microbes are dynamic organisms that rapidly adapt to their environment. Almost all of these adaptations are produced by genetic changes called mutations. Many bacteria have acquired mutant genes that protect them from antibiotics. This means that the same antibiotics that once killed a particular kind of bacteria now have no effect. This growing problem is encouraging scientists to try to create more vaccines to combat disease. Vaccines are preferred over antibiotics because they use the body's natural defenses to fight off the disease; moreover, it is less likely that bacteria will become resistant to vaccine treatments. But even vaccines can't prevent disease if people do not have access to them, as is often the case in poor communities and countries all over the world. To solve this problem, scientists are developing "edible vaccines."

As the name implies, these vaccines are taken in with the normal diet. Researchers have recently genetically altered crop plants to produce vaccines against certain diseases. The first edible vaccine was used for treating diseases that cause diarrhea in cattle. Vaccine genes were placed in potatoes that were then made into cattle feed. The edible vaccine worked as well as the shots normally given by veterinarians to treat these diarrheal diseases. Trials are under way to develop edible vaccines to treat similar diarrheal diseases in humans in Africa and Asia, where many children die each year from such diseases. So far, this novel type of vaccination seems to be working. Someday, scientists hope to produce foods that can vaccinate against many common ailments, including gonorrhea.

consequences—including unplanned pregnancy and sexually transmitted diseases—are not often depicted in a realistic fashion. However, when the media do present educational information about sexuality, adolescents and adults have been found to be receptive to the information.

Research shows that adolescents with close, warm, supportive relationships with their parents are more likely to postpone sexual intercourse, to limit the number of partners they have, and to effectively use contraception when they do become sexually active. Open discussion of sexual matters in homes, schools, and communities may assist in the prevention of gonorrhea and other STDs, as the experience of other countries that use these techniques has shown. These open discussion patterns improve communication between sexual partners, between parents and children, and between clinicians and patients. Better communication and understanding is essential if we hope to have any chance of eventually eliminating gonorrhea as a global health problem.

Abstinence—A strategy for preventing sexually transmitted diseases that centers on postponing sexual involvement.

Antibiotics—Drugs that kill or inhibit the growth of bacteria.

Antibodies—Protein molecules produced by the immune system as a protection against future disease.

Antigen—A substance that, when introduced into the body, stimulates the production of antibodies.

Anus—The opening of the rectum through which fecal matter is passed out of the body.

Asymptomatic—Showing no obvious signs or symptoms of a disease.

Bacterium (plural is *bacteria*)—Single-celled organism that multiplies by cell division and can cause disease in humans.

Bloodletting—A medical healing technique used since medieval times in which the infected patient is cut and some of the blood drained, because physicians often believed that "bad blood" was poisoning the body.

Cervical secretions—Fluid substances that are released from the cervix, often to help lubricate the vagina or as part of the menstrual cycle.

Cervix—The opening at the lower part of the uterus, connecting the uterus to the vagina.

Commensal—Living within the body of a host organism without impairing or injuring the host.

Communicable disease—An illness that can be spread from one person to another through close contact, including sexual activity.

Condom—A thin rubber or latex sheath worn over the penis during sexual intercourse to prevent pregnancy or sexually transmitted diseases.

Culture media—Chemical substances used to grow microorganisms in a laboratory.

Cytokines—Small proteins that mediate and regulate immunity.

Cytoplasm—The fluid that makes up the inside of a cell and holds the nucleus or organelles, if they are present.

Deoxyribonucleic acid (**DNA**)—Any of the nucleic acids that serve as the molecular basis of heredity.

Disseminated gonorrhea infection (**DGI**)—The spread of gonorrhea to parts of the body beyond the genitourinary tract.

Glossary

Dormant—Inactive.

Dysuria—Burning during urination.

Ectopic pregnancy—A condition in which a fertilized egg begins to develop outside of the uterus (typically in a fallopian tube).

Endocarditis—Inflammation of the lining of the heart and its valves.

Enzyme—Any protein that helps carry out an organism's functions by performing chemical reactions needed for processes such as digestion and metabolism.

Epidemic—An outbreak of disease that occurs on a larger than expected scale among a particular population.

Epididymis—Duct that transports sperm from the testicle to the vas deferens, the tube connecting the testes with the urethra.

Epithelium—The covering of most internal and external surfaces of the body and its organs.

Genitourinary tract—The body system that includes the organs used for reproduction and for eliminating liquid wastes from the body.

Genotype—The genetic makeup, rather than the physical appearance, of an organism.

Germ theory—The belief put forth in the mid-19th century that diseases were caused by infectious particles called microbes (at that time called "germs").

Gonad—A reproductive gland (such as the ovary in females or testis in males) that produces the cells needed for reproduction (in the case of humans, the female egg and the male sperm).

Gonococcal ophthalmitis—A gonorrhea infection in the eyes.

Gonoccocal pharyngitis—A gonorrhea infection in the throat.

Gonorrhea—A sexually transmitted disease caused by the bacterium *Neisseria gonorrhoeae*.

Gram staining—Procedure that is used to classify types of bacteria.

Host—A living thing used by another organism as a place to live in and obtain nutrients.

Human immunodeficiency virus (HIV)—The virus that causes acquired immunodeficiency syndrome (AIDS).

Immunity—The ability to resist infection by a particular pathogen, which occurs as a result of having formed antibodies against that pathogen, either through vaccination or having had the disease and successfully eliminated it.

Incidence—The number of new cases of a disease among a given population during a specified period of time (usually one year).

Laparoscopy—Surgical procedure in which a tiny scope is inserted in the abdomen through a small incision, allowing direct visualization of the abdominal cavity.

Metabolism—The series of chemical reactions within a cell, including digestion and reproduction, that allows it to stay alive.

Microbes—Tiny living organisms, such as bacteria and protozoans.

Microbiology—The study of microscopic organisms such as bacteria, fungi, and protists.

Microorganisms—Living things that are too small to be seen without the aid of a microscope.

Mucopurulent—Containing both mucus and pus.

Mucous membrane—A moist, mucus-covered tissue that lines the digestive, respiratory, reproductive, and urinary systems of the body.

Mucus—A sticky material made up of carbohydrates and other substances.

Neisseria gonorrhoeae—The bacterium that causes gonorrhea.

Pathogen—An organism that causes disease in another organism; in the past, pathogens were often referred to as "germs."

Pelvic inflammatory disease (PID)—An infection of the upper genital tract that is a serious and common complication of gonorrhea among women.

Penicillin—The first discovered antibiotic, and the first effective treatment for gonorrhea; it is derived from the fungus *Penicillium* and is effective in killing many types of bacteria and preventing bacterial growth.

Perineum—The area between the rectum and the external genital region.

Phenotype—The observable physical or biochemical characteristics of an organism, as determined by both genetic makeup and environmental influences.

Pili—Hair-like appendages on the surface of the *Neisseria gonorrhoeae* cell.

Glossary

Portal of entry—The site where a microorganism gets inside the body to start an infection.

Protozoan—A single-celled animal.

Purulent—Containing or causing the production of pus, a fluid product of inflammation.

Quinolones—Antibiotics that are effective against many forms of bacteria; they are very potent but can have side effects, including rare cases of tendon damage.

Rectum—The end portion of the intestine, attached to the anus.

Ribonucleic acid (RNA)—Any nucleic acid that contains ribose and uracil as part of its structure and plays a role in the chemical activities of a cell.

Safer sex—A strategy for preventing sexually transmitted diseases that focuses on promoting the use of condoms for all sexual activity.

Semen—The fluid produced by the male reproductive system that contains the sperm needed to fertilize the female egg to start a pregnancy.

Sexually transmitted disease (STD)—Any communicable disease spread through sexual intercourse or genital contact.

Spermicide—A contraceptive agent that kills sperm.

Urethra—The thin tube that carries urine from the bladder to the outside of the body.

Urethritis—Inflammation of the urethra.

Vaccination—The introduction of killed or weakened pathogens into the body to provoke an immune response that will provide immunity to the disease the pathogen causes.

Vectors—Organisms or objects that are able to carry a disease from one host to another.

Virus—An infectious agent that can replicate itself only within the cells of living hosts.

Bibliography

BOOKS AND ARTICLES

Bardin, T. "Gonococcal Arthritis." *Best Practice & Research Clinical Rheumatology* 17(2) 2003: 201–208.

Bauman, R. *Microbiology.* San Francisco: Pearson Education, 2002.

Branch, Shirley T. *Teaching the Facts About Gonorrhea.* Petersburg, VA: Virginia State University, 1981.

Braverman, P. K. "Sexually Transmitted Diseases in Adolescents." *Medical Clinics of North America* 84(4) (2000): 869–889.

Burstein, G. R., and K. A. Workowski. "Sexually Transmitted Diseases Treatment Guidelines." *Current Opinion in Pediatrics* 15(4) (2003): 391–397.

Cates, J. R., and W. Cates. "STD Prevention in the United States. Lessons from History for the New Millennium." *American Journal of Preventative Medicine* 16(1) (1998): 75–77.

Diamond, Jared. *Guns, Germs, and Steel: The Fates of Human Societies.* New York: W. W. Norton and Company, 1997.

Dicker, L. W., D. J. Mosure, R. Steece, and K. M. Stone. "Laboratory Tests Used in US Public Health Laboratories for Sexually Transmitted Diseases, 2000." *Sexually Transmitted Diseases* 31(5) (2004): 259–264.

Dolman, Claude E., and Richard J. Wolfe. *Theobald Smith, Microbiologist.* Boston: Boston Medical Library, 2003.

Farhat, S. E., M. Thibault, and R. Devlin. "Efficacy of a Swab Transport System in Maintaining Viability of *Neisseria gonorrhoeae* and *Streptococcus pneumoniae.*" *Journal of Clinical Microbiology* 39(8) (2001): 2958–2960.

Ford, C. A., J. Jaccard, S. G. Millstein, C. I. Viadro, J. L. Eaton, and W. C. Miller. "Young Adults' Attitudes, Beliefs, and Feelings about Testing for Curable STDs Outside of Clinic Settings." *Journal of Adolescent Health* 34(4) (2004): 266–269.

Garcia-De La Torre, I. "Advances in the Management of Septic Arthritis." *Rheumatic Disease Clinics of North America* 29 (2003): 61–75.

Gonorrhea: A Medical Dictionary, Bibliography, and Annotated Research Guide to Internet References. San Diego: ICON Health, 2004.

Guidance for Industry: Uncomplicated Gonorrhea—Developing Antimicrobial Drugs for Treatment. Washington, D.C.: U.S. Department of Health and Human Services, Food and Drug Administration, Center for Drug Evaluation and Research, 1998.

Bibliography

Hagen, Ronald A. *What You Always Wanted to Know About Safe Sex and STD's*. San Jose, CA: Writers Club Press, 2001.

Hethcote, Herbert W., and James A. Yorke. *Gonorrhea Transmission Dynamics and Control*. New York: Springer-Verlag, 1984.

Holmes, King K., P. Frederick Sparling, Per-Anders Mardh, Stanley M. Lemon, Walter E. Stamm, Peter Piot, and Judith N. Wasserheit. *Sexually Transmitted Diseases*. New York: McGraw-Hill Professional, 1998.

Levenson, D. "Increasing Cases of Drug-resistant Gonorrhea Prompt New CDC Treatment Recommendations for Gay and Bisexual Men." *Report on Medical Guidelines & Outcomes Research* 15(10) (2004): 8–9.

Mehaffey, P. C., S. D. Putnam, M. S. Barrett, and R. N. Jones. "Evaluation of in vitro Spectra of Activity of Azithromycin, Clarithromycin, and Erythromycin Tested Against Strains of *Neisseria gonorrhoeae* by Reference Agar Dilution, Disk Diffusion, and Etest Methods." *Journal of Clinical Microbiology* 34(2) (2002): 479–481.

Moran, J. "Gonorrhoea." *Clinical Evidence* (8) (2002): 1633–1641.

Nester, Eugene, et al. *Microbiology: A Human Perspective*, 3rd ed. New York: McGraw-Hill, 2001.

Nowicki, S., R. Selvarangan, and G. Anderson. "Experimental Transmission of *Neisseria gonorrhoeae* from Pregnant Rat to Fetus." *Infective Immunology* 67(9) (1999): 4974–4976.

Pavletic, A. J., P. Wolner-Hanssen, J. Paavonen, S. E. Hawes, and D. A. Eschenbach. "Infertility Following Pelvic Inflammatory Disease." *Infectious Diseases in Obstetrics and Gynecology* 7 (1999): 145–152.

Ross, J. D. "Systemic Gonococcal Infection." *Genitourinary Medicine* 72 (1996): 404–407.

Ross, Linda M., and Peter Dressler. *Sexually Transmitted Diseases Sourcebook*. Detroit: Omnigraphics, 1997.

Sarwal, S., T. Wong, C. Sevigny, and L. K. Ng. "Increasing Incidence of Ciprofloxacin-resistant *Neisseria gonorrhoeae* Infection in Canada." *Canadian Medical Association Journal* 168(7) (2003): 872–873.

Seeley, R. R., T. D. Stephans, and P. Tate. *Essentials of Anatomy and Physiology*. New York: WCB McGraw-Hill, 1999.

Shafer, M. A., J. Moncada, C. B. Boyer, K. Betsinger, S. D. Flinn, and J. Schachter. "Comparing First-void Urine Specimens, Self-collected Vaginal Swabs, and Endocervical Specimens to Detect *Chlamydia trachomatis* and

Neisseria gonorrhoeae by a Nucleic Acid Amplification Test." *Journal of Clinical Microbiology* 41(9) (2003): 4395–4399.

Shier, D., J. Butler, and R. Lewis. *Essentials of Human Anatomy and Physiology.* New York: McGraw-Hill, 2000.

Tapsall, J. "The Biology of *Neisseria gonorrhoeae*: A Model of Adaptation and Survival." *Venereology* 13(2) (2000): 63–69.

———. "Current Concepts in the Management of Gonorrhea." *Expert Opinion in Pharmacotherapy* 3(2) (2002): 147–157.

Thompson, E. C., and D. Brantley. "Gonoccocal Endocarditis." *Journal of the National Medical Association* 88(6) (1995): 353–356.

Tilden, J. H. *Gonorrhea and Syphilis—1912: A Drugless Treatment of Venereal Diseases.* Whitefish, MT: Kessinger Publishing Company, 1998.

Tramont, E. C. "Gonococcal Vaccines." *Clinical Microbiology Review* 2(Suppl) (2002): S74–S77.

Wolday, D., Z. Gebremariam, Z. Mohammed, W. Dorigo-Zetsma, H. Meles, T. Messele, A. Geyid, E. Sanders, and S. Maayan. "The Impact of Syndromic Treatment of Sexually Transmitted Diseases on Genital Shedding of HIV-1." *AIDS* 18(5) (2004): 781–785.

INTERNET RESOURCES

Advocates for Youth
http://www.advocatesforyouth.org
Established in 1980 as the Center for Population Options, Advocates for Youth champions efforts to help young people make informed and responsible decisions about their reproductive and sexual health.

The Center for Adolescent Health and the Law
http://www.cahl.org
The Center for Adolescent Health and the Law supports legislation and policies that promote the health of adolescents and their access to comprehensive health care.

Centers for Disease Control and Prevention (CDC)
http://www.cdc.gov
Official Website of the U.S. Centers for Disease Control and Prevention.

Emedicine.com
http://www.emedicine.com
The largest and most current clinical knowledge base available to physicians and health professionals.

Bibliography

4GirlsHealth

http://www.4girls.gov

Sponsored by the National Women's Health Information Center of the U.S. Department of Health and Human Services, this site was created to help girls ages 10–16 learn about health, growing up, and issues they may face. It focuses on health topics that girls are concerned about and helps motivate them to choose healthy behaviors by using positive, supportive, and nonthreatening messages. *4women.gov* is the adult version of this program.

Health A to Z

http://www.healthatoz.com

Includes information on a wide variety of health issues, including STDs. Perform a search on "gonorrhea" to find specific information related to this topic.

Cefrey, Holly. *Syphilis and Other Sexually Transmitted Diseases.* New York: Rosen Publishing Group, 2002.

Diamond, Jared. *Guns, Germs, and Steel: The Fates of Human Societies.* New York: W. W. Norton and Company, 1997.

Dolman, Claude E., and Richard J. Wolfe. *Theobald Smith, Microbiologist.* Boston: Boston Medical Library, 2003.

Nester, Eugene, et al. *Microbiology: A Human Perspective*, 3rd ed. New York: McGraw-Hill, 2001.

Parker, James M., and Philip M. Parker. *The Official Patient's Sourcebook on Gonorrhea: A Revised and Updated Directory for the Internet Age.* San Diego: ICON Health, 2002.

Shier, D., J. Butler, and R. Lewis. *Essentials of Human Anatomy and Physiology.* New York: McGraw-Hill, 2000.

Tilden, J. H. *Gonorrhea and Syphilis—1912: A Drugless Treatment of Venereal Diseases.* Whitefish, MT: Kessinger Publishing Company, 1998.

Websites

American Social Health Association
http://www.ashastd.org/stdfaqs/gonorrhea.html

Centers for Disease Control and Prevention
http://www.cdc.gov

Coalition for Positive Sexuality
http://www.positive.org/JustSayYes/stds.html

Diagnose Me.com
http://www.diagnose-me.com

Health Matters
http://www.niaid.nih.gov/factsheets/stdgon.htm

Kaiser Family Foundation
http://www.kff.org/

MedlinePlus
http://www.medlineplus.gov/

Sexual Health Information Center
http://reliance3.securesites.net/std/

Index

Index

Semen, 9, 102
Sexual behavior, media messages on, 96, 98
Sexual contact, in STD transmission, 9, 37, 47
Sexually transmitted disease (STD), 102
  early medical beliefs, 22–23
  history, 14, 21
  outbreaks of, 21, 81–82
  risk factors, 84
  specific diseases, 14–19
Sexual promiscuity, 20, 83–85, 95
Skin
  as barrier to infection, 34
  commensal bacteria of, 31–32
Skin rash, 78, 79
Smallpox, 6, 7, 82
Social risk factors, 88, 90
Spermicide, 22, 102
Spread. *See* Transmission
STD. *See* Sexually transmitted disease

Sterility. *See* Infertility
Stomach ulcers, 31
Substance abuse, 84
Sucrose test, 62
Superoxol test, 62–63
Symptoms, 9, 11–12, 49–54, 77–78
Syphilis, 18–19, 22–23, 45, 91

T cells, 36, 44
Teens. *See* Adolescents
Tests, diagnostic, 57–64
Transmission, 9, 37, 47–48
Treatment
  alternative medicine, 78
  antibiotics in, 12, 26, 68–72
  history of, 24–28
Treponema pallidum, 18
Trichomonas vaginalis, 19
Trichomoniasis, 19

Ultraviolet (UV) light in mutations, 33
Urethra, 9, 10, 102

Urethral lavage, 24–25
Urethritis, 52, 56, 102
UV light in mutations, 33

Vaccination, 94–95, 97, 102
Vagina, 9, 10
Vaginal yeast infection, 32, 45
Vectors, 47–48, 102
Viral STD, 15–18
Virus, 30, 102

White blood cells, 33, 34, 36, 43–44
Women
  incidence in, 83, 85
  portal of entry, 42
  symptoms, 11–12, 52
World Health Organization (WHO), 81, 82
World War II, 21, 27, 68–69

Yeast, vaginal, 32, 45

Picture Credits

10: © Peter Lamb
11: © Dr. David M. Phillips/Visuals Unlimited
15: © Dr. David M. Phillips/Visuals Unlimited
17: © Dr. Ken Greer/Visuals Unlimited
20: © Stefano Bianchetti/CORBIS
25: Courtesy the National Library of Medicine
35: © Peter Lamb
37: Courtesy the Public Health Image Library (PHIL), CDC
42: © Peter Lamb
50: Courtesy PHIL, CDC

54: Courtesy PHIL, CDC
60: © Raymond B. Otero/Visuals Unlimited
61: Courtesy PHIL, CDC
64: Courtesy PHIL, CDC
69: Courtesy PHIL, CDC
77: From STD Surveillance 2003, CDC
79: Courtesy PHIL, CDC
85: From STD Surveillance 2003, CDC
86: From STD Surveillance 2003, CDC
87: From STD Surveillance 2003, CDC

Cover: © Dr. David M. Phillips/Visuals Unlimited

About the Authors

Linda Kollar is a pediatric nurse practitioner and director of clinical services for the Division of Adolescent Medicine at Cincinnati Children's Hospital Medical Center in Cincinnati, Ohio. She did her undergraduate studies at the University of Cincinnati, College of Nursing, and received her Masters of Science in Nursing from Indiana University. She provides primary health care to a large population of adolescents in Cincinnati. Her research interests are related to adolescent sexual health. She has written for numerous nursing and medical textbooks and journals. She speaks about a broad range of adolescent health topics around the country. She has spent her entire nursing career working with and advocating for the health-care needs of adolescents.

Brian R. Shmaefsky is a professor of biology and environmental sciences at Kingwood College near Houston, Texas. He did his undergraduate studies in biology in Brooklyn, New York, and completed masters and doctoral studies at Southern Illinois University at Edwardsville. His research emphasis is in environmental physiology. Dr. Shmaefsky has many publications on science and education, some appearing in *American Biology Teacher* and the *Journal of College Science Teaching*. He regularly consults on general biology and microbiology textbook projects. Dr. Shmaefsky is also very active serving on environmental awareness and policy committees in Texas. He has two children, Kathleen and Timothy, and lives in Kingwood with his dog, Dusty.

About the Editor

The late **I. Edward Alcamo** was a Distinguished Teaching Professor of Microbiology at the State University of New York at Farmingdale. Alcamo studied biology at Iona College in New York and earned his M.S. and Ph.D. degrees in microbiology at St. John's University, also in New York. He had taught at Farmingdale for over 30 years. In 2000, Alcamo won the Carski Award for Distinguished Teaching in Microbiology, the highest honor for microbiology teachers in the United States. He was a member of the American Society for Microbiology, the National Association of Biology Teachers, and the American Medical Writers Association. Alcamo authored numerous books on the subjects of microbiology, AIDS, and DNA technology as well as the award-winning textbook *Fundamentals of Microbiology*, now in its sixth edition.

114